Advance Praise for *What to Feed Your Baby*

"Food, glorious food! Dr. Tanya is an experienced pediatrician and mom and she knows exactly how to get your baby to eat well and happily. *What to Feed Your Baby* provides easy, fun, and tasty advice!"

—Harvey Karp, M.D., F.A.A.P., author of *The Happiest Toddler on the Block* and *The Happiest Baby on the Block*

"Read it, do it, and watch your baby feel it. Writing from the experienced plate of a mother and pediatrician, Dr. Tanya helps parents shape young tastes toward lifelong healthy eating habits."

—William Sears, M.D., author of *The Baby Book*

"*What to Feed Your Baby* is the perfect mash-up: equal parts parenting handbook, developmental primer, cookbook, and personal experience. While Dr. Tanya's advice is focused on kids, the book is packed with great nutrition information for the entire family."

—Cara Natterson, M.D., *New York Times* bestselling author of *The Care and Keeping of You 1: The Body Book for Younger Girls*

"As a pediatrician I spend more time answering questions about feeding than any other topic. Dr. Tanya Altmann provides real-world advice on how to feed infants and children a healthy diet to ensure their optimal growth and development. As a doctor I'm going to be referring a lot of parents to this book, and as a dad I'm going to be trying out some of Dr. Tanya's tips in my own home!"

—David L. Hill, M.D., F.A.A.P., author of *Dad to Dad: Parenting Like a Pro*

"*What to Feed Your Baby* offers practical and tasty ways to build a foundation of healthy eating habits for the entire family. A must-read for all parents!"

—Ari Brown, M.D., pediatrician and author of the Baby 411 book series

"Healthy living starts with healthy eating, and the earlier we can teach our kids to eat well, the more likely they will grow up loving nutritious food. Dr. Tanya gives parents all the information they need to create healthy eating habits that will last a lifetime."

—Harley Pasternak, M.S.c., *New York Times* bestselling author of *The Body Reset Diet*

"Feeding your baby and toddler and all that encompasses—nutrition, eating behaviors, allergies—can be tricky business, bringing many a parent to her knees. Dr. Tanya Altmann has hit a homerun with *What to Feed Your Baby*. Answering even the questions you didn't know you had, it will be your go-to resource for navigating this often challenging aspect of child raising."

—Betsy Brown Braun, child development and behavior specialist and author of *Just Tell Me What to Say*

"Few things are as important to parents as teaching their children to eat right. Dr. Tanya Altmann's new book is packed with important information. It's a great read for worried parents, and everyone—no matter how much they already know—will be able to open this book and learn something new."

—Dina Rose, Ph.D., author of *It's Not About the Broccoli: Three Habits to Teach Your Kids for a Lifetime of Healthy Eating*

"Dr. Tanya helps parents make sense of early childhood nutrition and the newest feeding guidelines, and she teaches how to help children have a healthy relationship with food. I love the chapter on raising vegetarian and vegan kids, and I will have this informative, fun book within reach at all times!"

—Dr. Jenn Berman Mann, author of *SuperBaby: 12 Ways to Give Your Child a Head Start in the First 3 Years* and host of *VH1 Family Therapy with Dr. Jenn*

"*What to Feed Your Baby* whips together equal portions of facts and kid-friendly recipes for parents hoping to raise healthy eaters. Dr. Tanya's recommendations and list of Eleven Foundation Foods provide an easy-to-follow guide for parents looking for advice and feeding schedules to help even the pickiest kids. This is a must-have book for every family's dinner table!"

—Jennifer Shu, M.D., coauthor of *Heading Home with Your Newborn* and *Food Fights*

What to Feed YOUR BABY

A Pediatrician's Guide to the **Eleven Essential Foods** to Guarantee Veggie-Loving, No-Fuss, Healthy-Eating Kids

TANYA ALTMANN M.D., F.A.A.P.

with BETH SALTZ M.P.H., R.D.

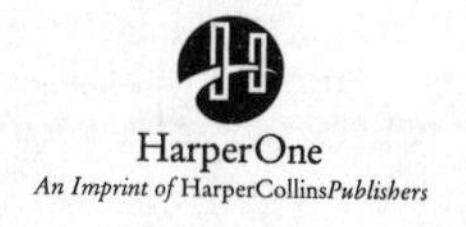

HarperOne
An Imprint of HarperCollins*Publishers*

This book is dedicated to my Papa, Dr. George Collen, the best role model for healthy eating.

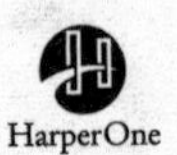

HarperOne

This book contains advice and information relating to health care for children. It is not intended to replace medical advice and should be used to supplement rather than replace regular care by your child's pediatrician. Since every child is different, you should consult your child's pediatrician on questions specific to your child.

While certain sections of the book contain advice for dealing with emergencies when a doctor is not available, it is recommended that you seek your child's pediatrician's advice whenever possible and that you consult with him or her before embarking on any medical program or treatment.

FIRST EDITION

Designed by Ralph Fowler

Library of Congress Cataloging-in-Publication Data
Names: Remer Altmann, Tanya, author.
Title: What to feed your baby : a pediatrician's guide to the eleven essential foods to guarantee veggie-loving, no-fuss, healthy-eating kids / Tanya Altmann.
Description: First edition. | New York, NY : HarperOne, 2016.
Identifiers: LCCN 2015033614 | ISBN 9780062404947 (paperback) | ISBN 9780062404930 (e-book)
Subjects: LCSH: Infants—Nutrition. | Food habits. | BISAC: FAMILY & RELATIONSHIPS / Parenting / General.
Classification: LCC RJ216 .R46 2016 | DDC 649/.3—dc23 LC record available at http://lccn.loc.gov/2015033614

16 17 18 19 20 RRD(H) 10 9 8 7 6 5 4 3 2 1

Contents

Introduction

Welcome to the Family Table

If you're reading this book, congratulations on entering the exciting world of parenting a beautiful new baby, toddler, or preschooler. I'm sure that you want to give your little one the best care possible. You probably ate healthy foods and took care of yourself during pregnancy, read the must-have pregnancy books, subscribed to the top parenting magazines and blogs, and organized your home in the safest way for your new child. What parent doesn't want the best for his or her child? Yet when it comes to food, many parents go about it all wrong.

I wrote *What to Feed Your Baby* after fifteen years of working with families in my pediatric practice—and raising my own kids. In my practice, I discuss the nutrients babies need to grow and develop, and I help parents decide when and how to start feeding solids; later, I discuss eating habits in older infants, toddlers, and children. I spend a good portion of each visit reviewing what kids eat and offering ways to make food more nutritious and appealing. Through my experience I have learned what it takes to raise a healthy, nonpicky, nutrition-loving child. And here's the key: *nutrition is critical to good health—and healthy eating starts when kids are under four, the younger the better.*

Unfortunately, much of the wisdom out there is confusing at best and destructive at worst. There are so many books, feeding trends, and blogs giving differing advice that most parents don't know where to turn. The parents who come to my office have witnessed dramatic changes in feeding recommendations over the years, leaving most of them confused and searching for the best way to nourish their young child. Currently, there is no "go-to feeding guide" that is truly authoritative, nor is there a medically endorsed feeding schedule for parents to follow. Lacking clear guidelines and succinct recommendations on what to feed infants and toddlers, parents struggle to understand the latest recommendations regarding introducing veggies, fruit, whole grains, lean proteins, dairy, and water into their child's diet. They crave an evidence-based feeding schedule with specifics on food portions, timing, and frequency.

Adding to the confusion, the latest medical recommendations about starting solids say . . . there are no longer any official recommendations! I can summarize current medical infant feeding recommendations in one sentence: "Feed whatever you want around six months as long as it isn't raw honey or a choking hazard." Not only is this information new, it's a little scary for many parents, who worry about food allergies, potential arsenic in rice cereal, the conundrum of starting with fruits versus veggies, waiting days between new foods, introducing table foods, exposure to pesticides and GMOs, and choking hazards. It's no wonder that parents are searching for guidance on what, when, and how to feed their baby!

As a pediatrician, author, mom, and spokesperson for the American Academy of Pediatrics, I have come up with a program that follows the safest, best practices for how to feed your baby and young child so that he or she eats and enjoys healthy, nutritious, delicious food. It's important to get specific nutrition in early, not only for the best brain development and growth, but also to train young taste buds and cultivate palates to enjoy and desire the healthiest of real, nonprocessed foods.

My program introduces eleven basic, building-block foods that should make up your child's diet. I call these the Eleven Foundation Foods. Many are foods that you're planning on feeding your baby or that your toddler or preschooler already loves. A few are surprises (for example, prunes and eggs), but I'll explain why your child needs to be eating and enjoying them. Feeding your child shouldn't take hours of research or a library full of books; it should be—and it is!—intuitive and easy. Learning about these Eleven Foundation Foods will save you time, money, and the headache that often goes into meal planning.

In part 1 of this book, I will unpack these Eleven Foundation Foods, explaining why they are important for your child's nutrition, and offer tips on how to introduce them to your child. *What* foods you choose is important, but equally important is *when* you introduce certain foods, flavors, and textures, as well as *how* you feed your child. So in part 2 I'll show you the *when* and *how,* including what you should be feeding your children based on their age and stage. Best of all, I'll show you how to get your kids to actually *eat* what you serve. No more picky eaters! The third part of the book will answer feeding FAQs: I'll present the most up-to-date, medically approved information on topics such as food allergies, vegetarian kids, navigating the organic and non-GMO aisles, and which trendy feeding plans to avoid. Lastly, I will include recipes created by my go-to dietitian and chef, Beth Saltz, R.D., to make meal planning even easier (and the results even tastier).

My hope is that as you read you'll see how simple it is to feed your kids nutritious food, to have happier mealtimes with your little ones, and to create healthy habits that stick with kids for life. If you follow the Eleven Foundation Foods Program, I believe you'll find the first five years of feeding easy instead of difficult, pleasant instead of joyless, and organized instead of haphazard. I have yet to meet a parent who doesn't want the absolute best for his or her child. Yet when it comes to food, some parents find themselves losing the battle. *What to Feed Your Baby* will ensure that your broccoli-loving baby doesn't become a toddler on an all-beige diet. You will be able to prevent your preschooler from a nightly plea for pasta. This book will arm you with the knowledge to help guard your family against the endless parade of tempting junk that kids demand. Not only will this book give you the absolute *best* food for your kids, it will also provide a real-world plan to get your kids (and your entire family) to eat and enjoy healthy foods *for life.*

PART ONE

Getting Started with the Eleven Foundation Foods Program

1.

The Eleven Foundation Foods

If you're a parent, you know that getting your kid to "eat healthily"—that is, to eat nutritious foods that will make him or her healthy—isn't always easy. In fact, meals can be a battle when your healthy food options turn mealtimes into meltdowns. I tell my patients that raising a healthy, nonpicky child who enjoys eating real, whole foods is quite simple. It comes down to this: start early with what I like to call the Eleven Foundation Foods.

If healthy choices are offered early and regularly to an infant (between six and twelve months), most children will quickly learn to accept (and even like!) them. There are many healthy foundation foods, even beyond my list of eleven, but I specifically chose the Eleven Foundation Foods after working with families in my office, studying nutrition, and examining child-feeding habits. I've found that the most effective time to introduce these foods is in the first six to twelve months, to establish healthy eating habits that ensure you'll have a great eater. If you're starting later, though, don't worry; it may take a bit longer, but you can still put your family on the right path. I have seen thousands of kids—from my own children to my patients—transform into healthy, nutrition-loving, nonpicky eaters by following this program. And you and *your* children can too!

The following section will introduce you to the Eleven Foundation Foods. For specifics on starting solids (when, where, how, and why) and how best to feed the Eleven Foundation Foods, just flip to chapter 2, "The Program."

Introducing the 11 Foundation Foods

Let's take a look at what it is about the Eleven Foundation Foods—eggs, prunes, avocados, fish, yogurt/cheese/milk, nuts and nut butters, chicken and/or beans/lentils, summer berries / winter citrus, green vegetables, whole grains, and water—that makes them so special.

1 Eggs

Eggs are a perfect single-ingredient food. Easy to prepare, they are a convenient and healthy source of protein, fat, and other nutrients, such as biotin and iron, which are important for growth and a healthy body. Eggs are a top source of protein for children, so introduce them early and frequently to your infant's diet. Research shows that eating a protein-rich breakfast can help your older child concentrate better in school and give him or her sustained energy. Furthermore, although it was once believed that eating eggs dangerously increased cholesterol levels, recent studies have demonstrated that this is not the case; it is perfectly healthy to eat eggs often.

Many parents ask me: Is it really safe to feed my infant a whole egg? My answer? Yes! You can feed your infant a whole egg (or rather, some portion of an egg that contains yolk plus white) starting at six months.

Previously it was recommended to start with egg yolks and wait to introduce egg whites, because the protein in the whites is potentially allergenic. Recent research has shown, however, that holding off on egg whites will not decrease your child's risk of becoming allergic; and current studies are examining whether early introduction of eggs into the diet of infants may actually decrease the likelihood of developing an allergy to eggs. (See chapter 8 for more information on food allergies.) If you introduce eggs early and serve them often, your child will accept them. Then you'll always have a very healthy morning (or anytime) option.

2 Prunes

Constipation is the most common tummy problem in infants and children. It occurs in babies as well as potty-training toddlers and older kids. Frustrated parents often respond by begging their kids to eat prunes or chasing them around with a bottle of stool softener—but this can be avoided by introducing prunes as a foundation food.

Prunes are fun fiber fruits that help resolve constipation likely because of their naturally occurring sorbitol—a form of sugar that is hard to absorb and can help soften stools. Prunes also have tons of important vitamins, minerals, and antioxidants—all this in a tiny, tasty, low-calorie package. An apple a day is important, but a prune a day works wonders to *prevent* constipation and keep young bodies healthy in the first place.

Use baby-food prunes regularly to treat and prevent constipation in infants. For older toddlers and children you can try whole prunes (also called dried plums), but cut them into small pieces. One prune a day is a great snack. If your child suffers from constipation, you can use pureed prunes as a mix-in with other foods, or up the amount of whole prunes to two or three (or even four) a day. Teach older toddlers that prunes (or dried plums) are yummy giant raisins—kids love that! Look for the prunes sold in cute little single-serve packages so fingers won't get sticky.

3 Avocados

Did you know that avocados are actually fruits? They are high in potassium, fiber, and healthy monounsaturated fat, which is good for hearts of all ages. Don't be discouraged if your infant doesn't immediately take to mashed avocado. Some foods must be introduced a dozen times before a child will take to them. Take photos of that funny face as your infant spits the avocado out—and keep trying. Most infants and kids will eventually enjoy avocados.

Many health-conscious parents offer avocado as their baby's first food. Whether you introduce it first or farther down the line, puree or fork-mash it for lumpier texture. As your infant grows, she will find small pieces of avocado fun to try to pick up and smash, and preschoolers can join their parents in enjoying guacamole.

4 Fish

Fish is a great natural source of protein. It also contains vitamin D—a vitamin that most kids (and adults too!) need more of. Vitamin D is important for building bones, preventing illness, and lowering the risk of certain diseases, including cancer. The oils in fatty fish such as salmon are high in omega-3 fatty acids, especially EPA and DHA, which are great for brain and eye development and thus are especially important for pregnant women, infants, and young children. Other good fish sources of EPA and DHA include mackerel, bluefish, lake trout, and tuna.

Some adults dislike fish because, having never had it when they were little, they are unfamiliar with its taste and smell. By introducing fish early (any time after six months of age), you will help your children grow to enjoy fish and the important nutrition it provides throughout their life.

5 Yogurt, Cheese, and Milk

Dairy products are healthy for children and packed with a powerful punch of nine essential nutrients that most kids don't get enough of—

calcium, potassium, phosphorus, protein, vitamin A, vitamin D, vitamin B_{12}, riboflavin, and niacin. In fact, milk is the *best* source of vitamin D for kids, which, as mentioned above, is important for growing healthy bones, preventing illness, and lowering the risk of certain diseases (including cancer).

Although babies under one year of age should not drink regular cow's milk, yogurt and cheese can and should be introduced after six months of age. After one year, offer whole or reduced-fat cow's milk; toddlers need the nutrients and fat for brain development. Even if you are still nursing, offer sips of cow's milk to get your toddler used to the taste. For young ones over age two, nonfat or low-fat milk is best, since these offer the same nutrition but with less fat (milk fat being something that even *skinny* kids no longer need).

When choosing yogurt, try plain initially. If you decide to go for flavored yogurt, look for lower-sugar, no-fake-color options, with live or active cultures to keep kids' guts healthy and help boost immunity to prevent illness. Greek yogurt is also delicious and a great choice for any age, as it packs more protein per serving than does regular yogurt.

For cheese, infants tend to like mild-tasting options such as jack, mild cheddar, mozzarella, and cottage cheese. All these are good choices—just break or shred the cheese into tiny soft pieces.

6 Nuts and Nut Butters

Nuts and nut butters are delicious, healthy, and convenient. Nutrient-wise, they offer vegetarian protein, vitamin E, and healthy monounsaturated fats. Nuts and nut butters are an easy way to add healthy protein to any meal, even breakfast!

Start your older infants and children with creamy nut butter by itself or on whole-grain bread. Peanut butter and almond butter are favorites with young kids. Eventually your preschooler will be better able to handle chewing crunchy nut butters and small pieces of raw nuts—a great snack or portable protein to carry with you anywhere.

Some parents worry that kids will become allergic if they eat nuts too early. Research suggests that this is *not* true. (See chapter 8 on food allergies for more information.) The bottom line: introducing nuts early does not put your child at risk of becoming allergic, and studies are now showing that introducing earlier may better decrease the chances of later developing an allergy. So I recommend that parents introduce this important food early on.

7 Chicken and/or Beans/Lentils (Vegetarian Alternative)

Chicken and beans are healthy sources of protein and easy finger food for older infants and toddlers. The key is getting your children used to eating healthy, plain chicken at a young age. Countless children will consume chicken only if it's breaded, fried, and in a familiar oval shape. Chicken can taste great on its own, so get your kids used to grilled, baked, broiled, barbecued, poached, and sautéed preparations.

Infants need a source of iron and zinc around six months of age, and chicken is a great one. It can be pureed with a veggie to make a nutritious baby food, or cut into tiny pieces for little fingers to self-feed. At restaurants, just order a side of grilled chicken from the adult menu and cut a small portion into tiny pieces for your child.

For a vegetarian alternative or to add variety to your child's protein intake, introduce beans or lentils—basically, anything in the legume family. High in fiber, protein, vitamins, and minerals, legumes are versatile and inexpensive.

For infants, mash or puree cooked beans or lentils. For toddlers and preschoolers, offer beans alone, as well as mashed in a quesadilla or with a potato. Chickpeas tend to be a favorite in many families, especially in the form of hummus.

8 Summer Berries / Winter Citrus

All fruits are great, but seasonal berries and citrus in particular are packed with nutrition. Both are low in calories, are high in fiber, and contain vitamins and minerals your body needs to function normally and stay healthy.

In addition to fiber, berries contain loads of vitamin C and other antioxidants important for vision and brain development, as well as phytonutrients that may help protect against disease later on in life. Offer berries plain, in a smoothie, or as dessert. Buy berries fresh in the summer season, when you can. In the winter, when berries aren't in season, buy frozen! They have the same nutritional value, and you can easily add them to pancakes, yogurt, or smoothies.

During winter, when your immune system needs them most, citrus fruits are in season. Oranges and other citrus fruits are a fantastic source of many vitamins; they are high in vitamin C, folate, and fiber, all of which many kids need more of. Clementines (a cross between oranges and tangerines) are super-easy for kids to peel, are seedless, and can easily be packed in school lunches. Best of all, kids (and parents) love to eat them!

9 Green Vegetables

We all remember our parents telling us to eat our veggies, but I'll say it again. Attention parents: if *you* do not eat green vegetables, your children won't eat them either! But don't do it *just* for the kids. People who eat more green veggies are linked with lower disease rates and a healthier weight. Green veggies have almost every vitamin and mineral you can think of. Offer your children green veggies in any form—steamed, roasted, sautéed, raw, and in soups and salads (preparing and introducing them as suggested in chapter 2). Calorie for calorie, leafy greens such as kale, Swiss chard, and spinach pack more nutrition than any other food.

Green veggies are a great first food for babies, and they're easy to cook and then puree or fork-mash to the desired consistency. Add breast milk or water to thin the puree if needed. Try mixing pureed green vegetables with pureed chicken or orange veggies for a variety of flavors and colors.

Some green veggies may take multiple tries for your infant to accept, but that's okay. I promise that after two weeks of parental attempts, your baby will love them and grow to be a much healthier, nonpicky eater because of your persistence and commitment to her nutrition early on.

As your infant gets older, offer cut-up pieces of soft-cooked (steamed or boiled) vegetables such as broccoli, green beans, carrots, and sweet potatoes as finger foods—a variety of colors is great. Some toddlers will become picky, even after starting off liking veggies, and may go on a green veggie strike for a bit, but if you keep serving veggies, those same toddlers will grow to accept and enjoy veggies for life.

10 Whole Grains

Walk through the center aisles of the grocery store and you will see thousands of highly processed grain products. Most have very little fiber, very long ingredient lists, and added color. Try to make all of your grains, both for your children and for you, "whole"—meaning that the first ingredient listed should be "100 percent whole-grain wheat" (or another whole grain such as oats or quinoa).

Banning grains may be popular with some dieting adults, but grains are delicious and nutritious for children. You *should* include them in a child's diet. Even if your child has a food allergy, you can choose from many alternative grains. (See chapter 8 for more information on food allergies.) Whole grains are a great source of energy, provide fiber for a healthy digestive system, and feed the healthy bacteria in our intestines.

Look for at least 3 grams of fiber per serving for most grain-based foods.

11 Water

Most people should be drinking primarily water, and infants can start working toward that goal as soon as they start solid food. Even though breast milk is still providing most of your child's liquid and nutrition at six months, offering small sips of water starting around that age is a great way to get your infant used to the taste of plain water. Infants who like plain water grow into toddlers and young children who like plain water, and eventually into adults who like plain water.

This is important: no juice! Even diluted juice only gets kids used to the taste of sweet beverages. There's plenty of time for that when they get older. Start them off well now, and drinking water will become a lifelong healthy habit.

2.

The Program

Now that you know a bit about each of the Eleven Foundation Foods and why they provide important nutrition for your young child's growth and development, you may be wondering, "How exactly do I feed chicken to my six-month-old?" or "Can I really give a PB&J sandwich to my nine-month-old?" This chapter will explain when and how to introduce each of the Eleven Foundation Foods to your infant in the first year of life, as well as how to deliciously prepare them for toddlers, preschoolers, and the entire family.

A note before we begin. I've broken the program into three parts so that you can easily find the information you need based on the age of your child. The Infant Program is for children aged six to twelve months, the Toddler Program for those from one year of age until their third birthday, and the Preschooler Program for kids aged three to five. In each program, I'll suggest portion sizes and let you know how to present that particular food. You'll also find tips from my dietitian and chef, Beth Saltz, on how to use the grocery store to your advantage, notes on important safety considerations, and recipe ideas. When you're done, you should have a plan you can easily put together for how best to feed your children.

Infant Program: Ages Six Months to Twelve Months

Before six months of age, your baby should be drinking the best milk available. I strongly recommend breast milk (see chapter 3). Starting around six months of age, the goal is to have your child grow to enjoy all Eleven Foundation Foods over the subsequent six-month period so that she is regularly eating them all by one year of age. Chapters 4 through 6 provide sample meal and snack plans that integrate all the foundation foods by the appropriate age.

Liquid Measure Equivalents

1 cup = 8 ounces = 16 tablespoons = 240 milliliters

½ cup = 4 ounces = 8 tablespoons = 120 milliliters

¼ cup = 2 ounces = 4 tablespoons = 60 milliliters

⅛ cup = 1 ounce = 2 tablespoons = 30 milliliters

1 tablespoon = 3 teaspoons = 15 milliliters

Dry Measure Equivalents

½ cup = 8 tablespoons = 24 teaspoons

¼ cup = 4 tablespoons = 12 teaspoons

⅛ cup = 2 tablespoons = 6 teaspoons

1 tablespoon = 3 teaspoons

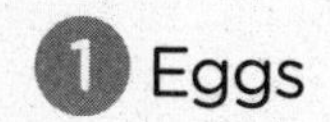

1 Eggs

1 large egg = about 3 tablespoons = about 1½ ounces

Age: Six to eight months

PORTION SIZE: 1 tablespoon (about one-third of a large cooked egg), two to three times per week

HOW TO SERVE: Puree or mash one hard-boiled or scrambled egg and serve. For a more liquid consistency, add breast milk or water to the pureed or mashed egg.

Age: Eight to twelve months

PORTION SIZE: 1 to 2 tablespoons (about half of a large cooked egg), two to three times per week

HOW TO SERVE: Scrambled eggs are a fantastic first finger food. They aren't too messy, and an eight- or nine-month-old can easily pick up the pieces. Most infants quickly enjoy the taste of a plain scrambled egg. You can also hard-boil and mash or cut the egg into small pieces.

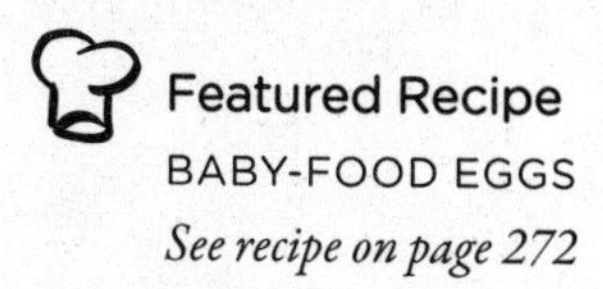

Featured Recipe

BABY-FOOD EGGS

See recipe on page 272

Cooking Help Desk

Stuck to the Pan? When cooking eggs, it's fine to add a little bit of real butter or healthy oil, such as olive or canola oil, to the pan so the eggs don't stick.

2 Prunes

Age: Four to six months

PORTION SIZE: 1 teaspoon to 1 tablespoon, three to seven times per week

HOW TO SERVE: Serve pureed.

Age: Six to eight months

PORTION SIZE: 1 to 2 tablespoons, three to seven times per week

HOW TO SERVE: You can feed baby-food prunes alone, or mix them with other fruits and vegetables or with infant cereals.

Age: Eight to twelve months

PORTION SIZE: 1 to 2 tablespoons, three to seven times per week

HOW TO SERVE: You can start to mix baby-food prunes with lumpier foods such as oatmeal. Many of my patients feed their infants oatmeal with prunes every morning for a healthy breakfast that keeps the babies regular.

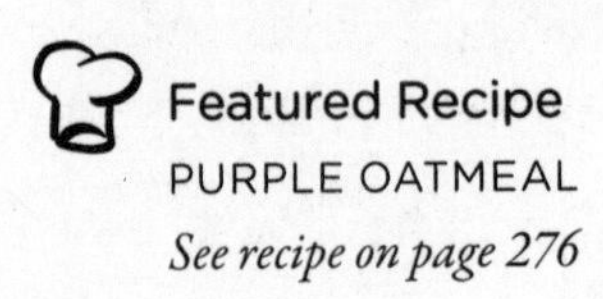

Featured Recipe

PURPLE OATMEAL

See recipe on page 276

3 Avocados

Age: Four to six months

PORTION SIZE: 1 teaspoon to 1 tablespoon, two to three times per week

HOW TO SERVE: Puree a bit of avocado and offer your baby a small spoonful. If she doesn't accept it, don't worry. She may not be ready for solids. Just wait a week or two and try again.

Age: Six to eight months

PORTION SIZE: 1 teaspoon to 1 tablespoon, two to three times per week

HOW TO SERVE: Puree or fork-mash a piece of avocado. Sliced avocado is easy to order on the side in a restaurant, giving you a healthy food to fork-mash and feed your baby while you enjoy your meal.

Don't be discouraged if your infant doesn't immediately take to mashed avocado. I have great photos of my older son making a funny face the first few times he tried it. Some foods must be introduced a dozen times before a child will take to them. Keep trying and most will eventually enjoy avocado—my boys now do.

Age: Eight to twelve months

PORTION SIZE: 1 to 2 tablespoons, two to three times per week

HOW TO SERVE: Diced pieces of avocado are fun for infants this age to try to pick up, squish, and self-feed. If you're introducing avocado for the first time at this age, don't be surprised if your little one makes a funny face. Keep trying, and soon he will accept and love avocado.

> ➢ Dr. Tanya's Tip: Too Fishy!
>
> **Soak fish in ice water for twenty minutes before cooking to decrease the fishy smell and taste. Rinse canned tuna in cold water for sandwiches that are less fishy-tasting.**

4 Fish

Age: Six to eight months

PORTION SIZE: 1 teaspoon to 1 tablespoon, one to two times per week

HOW TO SERVE: Thoroughly cook all fish. It's okay to season it lightly (with a little lemon, salt, or herbs) if your whole family will be sharing the fish. Puree or fork-mash the infant's portion very well and add a little moisture with water, breast milk, or chicken or vegetable broth. My eight-month-old preferred salmon mixed with pureed vegetables like carrots or sweet potatoes.

Age: Eight to twelve months

PORTION SIZE: 1 to 2 tablespoons (or more if desired), one to two times per week

HOW TO SERVE: Cook fish thoroughly. Light seasoning is okay (see above). If you are eating fish, feel free to offer your baby a

> **Safety Tip**
>
> **Fish Bones:** Smash or pull apart the fish well to ensure that there are no hidden fish bones, as even a tiny bone can be a potentially dangerous choking hazard for an infant.

piece of mashed fish off your plate. Avoid high-mercury fish such as swordfish and shark (see Safety Tip on fish and mercury on page 33). Add a little broth and/or pureed vegetables if needed to make the fish moister and tastier for your baby.

Featured Recipe

SALMON TWO WAYS (SIMPLE SALMON)

See recipe on page 297

➢ Dr. Tanya's Tip: Omega-3 Fatty Acids

Omega-3s are essential fatty acids, needed for our bodies to function normally. Some recent research suggests that an omega-rich diet may be associated with a reduced chance of asthma or wheezing, especially when omega-3s are introduced between six and twelve months of age.[1] Fish is one of the best sources of omega-3s available. Serve low-mercury fish to your whole family twice a week.

5 Yogurt, Cheese, and Milk

Age: Six to eight months (only yogurt at this stage)

PORTION SIZE: 1 ounce of yogurt (2 tablespoons), three to four times per week

HOW TO SERVE: My favorite way to introduce dairy in this age group is yogurt. Infants *love* yogurt. To them it's as good as ice cream! Choose a plain whole-milk yogurt (see Beth's Grocery Guide on page 21 for yogurt-buying tips) and feed it with a baby spoon. You can also mix plain yogurt with your own pureed prunes or other fruit such as Baby Food Strawberries, see recipe page 272.

Age: Eight to twelve months

PORTION SIZE:

Yogurt: 2 to 4 ounces, three to four times per week

Cheese: 1 1-inch cube (shred yourself or cut into small pieces)

HOW TO SERVE:

Yogurt: Give your older infant her own spoon to use, while you manage most of the feeding with your spoon.

Cheese: You can introduce small bite-size pieces of cheese as a snack or with any meal. Popular options at this age include mozzarella and cheddar.

➢ Dr. Tanya's Tip: Probiotics for Kids

Probiotics (aka a type of live microorganism or good gut bacteria), found in various dairy products, are beneficial for people of all ages, but especially babies born via C-section and infants not receiving breast milk. Babies born vaginally tend to have healthier gut flora due to all the stuff they ingested while passing through the birth canal.[2] In particular, anyone on antibiotics should take probiotics to help replace the good gut bacteria killed by their medication and to prevent overgrowth of bad bacteria in the gut.

Probiotics are found naturally in breast milk. Yogurt with live cultures and yogurt drinks such as kefir also contain probiotics, either naturally or as additives. Make sure your yogurt label reads, "contains live and active cultures." Certain probiotics (lactobacillus, for example) are also available in chewable, liquid, and powder forms.

Research shows that kids who take daily probiotics have fewer colds and illnesses during the winter months, miss fewer days of school, and use fewer antibiotics.[3] For these reasons, I think it would benefit everyone to take daily probiotics and/or eat yogurt with live cultures, especially during winter months and when on antibiotics.

Safety Tip

Cow's Milk: Babies under the age of one shouldn't drink regular cow's milk. Cow's milk does not supply proper nutrition for infants that young—it lacks iron and other nutrients found in breast milk—and it isn't as easily digested as breast milk. In addition, cow's milk does not contain the healthiest types of fat for growing babies, and it has too much protein and too much of certain minerals for a baby's immature kidneys to handle. Cow's milk can also irritate the lining of a baby's stomach and intestines and cause anemia.

BETH'S GROCERY GUIDE

Comparing Sugar Content in Yogurts

Brand A: Vanilla yogurt (4 ounces) = 17 grams sugar (about 4 teaspoons!)

Brand B: Vanilla baby yogurt (4 ounces) = 13 grams sugar (about 3 teaspoons)

Brand C: Greek "kid" yogurt (4 ounces) = 13 grams sugar (about 3 teaspoons)

Brand D: Plain yogurt (4 ounces) = 6 grams sugar (1½ teaspoons)

Food companies are not required to specify grams of *added* sugar on the label; they simply list *total* sugar. Remember that yogurt and milk already have their own healthy, natural sugar to start with. So to figure out how much sugar has been *added,* compare the plain to the flavored version (remembering to correct for equal serving sizes). Sound like a pain? Yes, it is. But the results are revealing. You can see above that Brand A has almost three times the amount of sugar as the plain version—not a good choice. Both Brands B and C would be fine. Better yet, stick with the plain yogurt and add your own fruit for flavor.

6 Nuts and Nut Butters

Age: Six to eight months

PORTION SIZE: ½ to 1 teaspoon, two to three times per week

HOW TO SERVE: Nutritionally, it's fine to give nut butter to an infant of this age; the problem is the stickiness and consistency, which make it hard for such a young infant to move the nut butter around in the mouth properly and safely. I like to melt a small amount into baby cereal such as oatmeal, making sure the mixture isn't too sticky and thick. Around eight months you can start to introduce creamy nut butter by itself, in an extremely thin layer on either your finger or a spoon for your infant to lick off.

Age: Eight to twelve months

PORTION SIZE: An extremely thin layer, two to three times per week

HOW TO SERVE: Spread a very thin layer on thinly sliced soft, whole-grain bread. Cut the bread into tiny pieces and observe as your older infant/toddler picks them up and eats them. Alternatively, he can lick the nut butter off the bread, a spoon, or your finger.

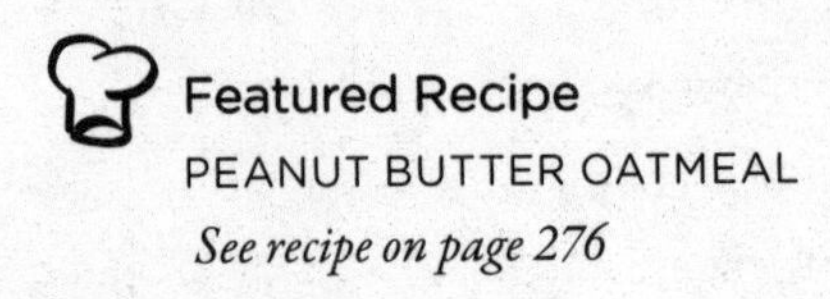

Featured Recipe

PEANUT BUTTER OATMEAL

See recipe on page 276

Safety Tip

Choking Hazard: Thick nut butter (or a glob of nut butter) can be a choking hazard, because it's hard for an infant to move around in his mouth and can easily get stuck on the top of the mouth or in the back of the throat or airway. Make sure that you use an extremely thin layer of creamy (not crunchy) nut butter—a layer so thin that you can still see the spoon or your finger through it—and watch your infant closely while he's eating.

7 Chicken and/or Beans/Lentils (Vegetarian Alternative)

Age: Six to eight months

PORTION SIZE: ½ to 1 tablespoon, two to three times per week

HOW TO SERVE: Both chicken and beans/lentils are fine for infants beginning around six months. Both should be cooked, then pureed. For chicken, you may need to add extra chicken or vegetarian broth to thin the puree out; alternatively, breast milk is fine as a thinner. For beans, you can quickly puree canned kidney, garbanzo, or white beans, thinning with broth or breast milk as needed. You can also use healthy homemade, strained chicken broth (or store-bought organic, low-sodium chicken broth) to mix with or to thin infant cereal, pureed veggies, or any baby food.

Age: Eight to twelve months

PORTION SIZE: 2 tablespoons, three to five times per week

HOW TO SERVE: Instead of pureeing chicken or beans/lentils, gradually adjust the texture to fork-mashed. After your baby gets used to the fork-mashed consistency, introduce very small bits of moist chicken or beans. Again, you can add liquid or pureed vegetables to achieve a moist, soft consistency. If the family dinner is chicken, you can now start putting very small pieces on your baby's tray. At restaurants you can order plain grilled chicken breast and shred a bit of it into very small pieces. At this age, beans/lentils can be a side dish at any meal. Fork-mash them or cut them into very small pieces for little fingers to pick up.

Featured Recipe

BABY-FOOD CHICKEN

See recipe on page 273

➢ Dr. Tanya's Tip: The Importance of Iron

Around six months of age, all infants need an additional source of iron in their diet (your pediatrician can let you know the exact amount depending on your child's age). The iron is needed to make red blood cells to deliver oxygen throughout the body during this period of rapid growth. Offering an iron-rich food daily will help provide your infant with the iron he needs. Good iron sources for young infants include red meat, poultry, fish, and fortified cereals, such as infant rice cereal.

Infants who were born early (that is, premature babies) need extra iron supplements even before six months of age and are usually placed on liquid iron supplements (or a liquid multivitamin with iron) to ensure that they receive enough iron for proper growth and development.

8 Summer Berries / Winter Citrus

Age: Six to eight months

PORTION SIZE: 1 to 2 tablespoons, two to three times per week

HOW TO SERVE: Give your infant pureed or mashed berries, alone or mixed with infant cereal, depending on the consistency your little one can handle. Try letting your infant suck on a clementine or orange wedge that you hold tightly, so he can't break off a piece.

Age: Eight to twelve months

PORTION SIZE: 2 tablespoons, two to three times per week (*Note:* Your infant should eat *some* type of fruit daily.)

HOW TO SERVE: Provide cut-up, soft berries or very small pieces of citrus, such as oranges or clementines.

Featured Recipe

BABY-FOOD STRAWBERRIES

See recipe on page 272

➢ Dr. Tanya's Tip: Finger-Food Feeding

Berries make a fun, nutritious, delicious finger food that infants love to gobble! Start by cutting blueberries in half, but in a few months your infant may be able to handle soft whole blueberries. Cut ripe strawberries and other berries into bite-size pieces perfect for little hands to pick up. My nine-month-old loves tiny pieces of raspberries. They are so soft they practically melt as he smashes them with his gums.

9 Green Vegetables

Age: Four to six months

PORTION SIZE: 1 to 2 tablespoons, one to two times per week

HOW TO SERVE: Pureed veggies are a great first food for babies. Simply steam or boil and then puree any green vegetable (or combination of vegetables). Add breast milk or water to thin the consistency until it's runny and soup-like. Green veggies that are especially easy to steam (or boil or sauté) and puree include peas, green beans, zucchini, spinach, broccoli, and asparagus.

Age: Six to eight months

PORTION SIZE: 2 tablespoons, two to three times per week

HOW TO SERVE: Puree or fork-mash soft-cooked veggies to the desired consistency. Add breast milk or water to thin the consistency if needed. Mix different vegetables together for a variety of flavors. My boys loved anything with baby-food carrots, so I mixed whatever they *didn't* seem to love with carrots and they ate it!

➢ Dr. Tanya's Tip: Beyond Green Veggies

You don't have to start green, because many infants love orange veggies (for example, carrots or sweet potatoes) and/or yellow veggies (for example, squash) as well. Any and all vegetables are healthy for infants and older children. It's a good idea, though, to introduce green veggies by around six months of age and continue offering them regularly, to ensure that your infant will grow into a toddler and older child who loves green veggies.

Age: Eight to twelve months

PORTION SIZE: 2 to 3 tablespoons, three to five times per week (*Note:* Your infant should eat *some* type of veggie daily.)

HOW TO SERVE: Offer cut-up small pieces of soft-cooked veggies as finger food. Infants love foods of pretty colors, so introduce veggies in a variety of colors and textures. Steam green beans, cut into small pieces, and let your child practice feeding herself.

Featured Recipe

BABY-FOOD BROCCOLI

See recipe on page 270

10 Whole Grains

Age: Four to six months

PORTION SIZE: 1 to 2 tablespoons infant cereal such as brown rice, oatmeal, barley, or quinoa, three to four times per week

HOW TO SERVE: Add breast milk or water as directed to make a very thin, soup-like consistency. If your infant doesn't take the cereal or pushes it out with his tongue, he may not yet be ready to start solids. Try again in a week or two.

Safety Tip

No Cereal in a Baby Bottle: Do not put cereal in your baby's bottle (unless advised by your pediatrician as a treatment for reflux). In general, adding cereal to a bottle is not a good or safe idea: the practice contributes to overfeeding, obesity, and choking (due to the thickness of the cereal). Furthermore, contrary to popular belief, it will not help a baby sleep through the night. Once your baby is truly ready to start cereal, he should be able to eat it from a spoon.

Age: Six to eight months

PORTION SIZE: 2 tablespoons infant cereal such as brown rice or oatmeal, increasing to 2 to 4 tablespoons as your infant grows, three to four times per week

HOW TO SERVE: When buying infant cereal, choose a whole-grain option such as brown rice, oatmeal, barley, or quinoa cereal. Add breast milk or water to make a liquid, soup-like consistency. You can gradually increase thickness from soup-like to slightly thicker as tolerated. Feel free to mix in pureed prunes, other fruits, or even veggies. As your baby becomes more experienced with eating, branch out from infant-specific cereal and try regular hot cereal, thinned with breast milk or extra water.

Age: Eight to twelve months

PORTION SIZE: ¼ slice soft, whole-grain bread, and/or 2 to 4 tablespoons whole-grain pasta, rice, or cereal, five to seven times per week

HOW TO SERVE: Choose whole-grain "O" cereal as a snack, rather than refined-grain puffed baby snacks. Try offering tiny pieces of healthy bread, breaking off a little bit at a time and placing it on your child's high-chair tray.

Featured Recipe

PEANUT BUTTER OATMEAL

See recipe on page 276

> ➢ Dr. Tanya's Tip: Whole-Grain Os
>
> **Whole-grain "O" cereals are a great finger food for infants. You can easily carry them around, and they are a healthier alternative than the "puffs" commonly consumed. Look for products with at least 3 grams of fiber per serving.**

➢ Dr. Tanya's Tip: Whole Grains

Try to make the grains your family eats "whole-grain." This is especially important for the grains your family consumes most often, such as cereal and bread. If the first ingredient listed on the label is "enriched flour," the product isn't whole-grain. Oatmeal is an easy and very healthy start to the day.

BETH'S GROCERY GUIDE

Buying Grain Products

While shopping for grains and grain products, look for items with *short* ingredient lists. You should be able to pronounce and hopefully identify all the ingredients. Avoid chemicals and additives.

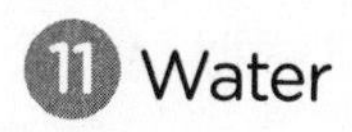

11 Water

Age: Six to eight months

PORTION SIZE: A few sips, daily as desired

HOW TO SERVE: Give your baby sips from a bottle or cup. Breast milk and solid foods are still providing most of your baby's hydration. Once you introduce solid food, introduce water with meals or throughout the day to get her used to the flavor and routine.

Age: Eight to twelve months

PORTION SIZE: 1 to 2 ounces at meals, daily

HOW TO SERVE: Offer water in a straw cup, sippy cup, or regular cup. As soon as possible, make water a routine at meals, snacks, and throughout the day.

Toddler Program: Ages One and Two

What's the most important difference between feeding infants and feeding toddlers? Many parents would say that infants eat pureed food while toddlers graduate to lumps and pieces. While this is true, the most important difference is that parents primarily give infants *special* food—food that the rest of the family isn't eating. The big goal of feeding toddlers should be their gradual progression to eating with the rest of the family.

My feeding program will enable you to respect the changing feeding stages of your toddler, while gradually moving toward whole-family meals.

I'll lay out the Eleven Foundation Foods Program as it applies to toddlers below, while in chapter 5 I'll tackle your toddler's specific feeding development and progression. Eating together as a family can be easy and fun!

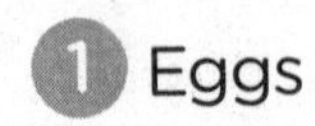

1 Eggs

Age: One and two years

PORTION SIZE: ½ to 1 egg, two to four times per week

HOW TO SERVE: You can start trying mixed egg dishes, like omelets or frittatas, which are a great way to get your child used to eating little bits of veggies with egg. A small amount of cheese added to the egg is fine too. French toast made with 100 percent whole-wheat bread, drenched in egg, is another delicious egg option. Serve in bite-size pieces.

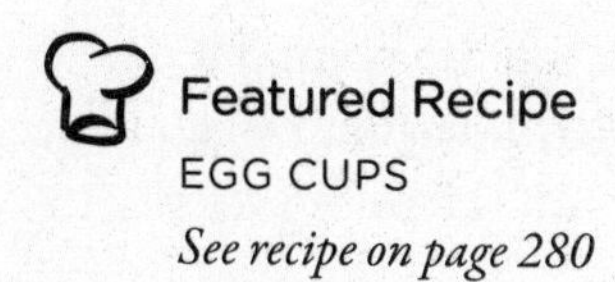

See recipe on page 280

Cooking Help Desk

Love Those Leftovers: Make extra scrambled egg, omelet, frittata, or even French toast. These are easy to reheat the next day (even in the microwave) for a quick breakfast or as a snack. I've also found, with my busy schedule, that it's helpful to make scrambled eggs or veggie egg scrambles at night and refrigerate them. After a quick reheat in the microwave, they offer my kids a healthy, quick breakfast the next morning (or even over the next few days).

➢ Dr. Tanya's Tip: Start Plain

Always serve French toast plain. Avoid adding powdered sugar or syrup. Toddlers will love it plain, so let them enjoy the real taste and don't let them get used to a super-sweet, sugary breakfast. Besides, it's less messy without the sticky syrup!

2 Prunes

Age: One and two years

PORTION SIZE: ½ to 1 prune, two to three times per week, or daily if needed

HOW TO SERVE: You can now try whole prunes (also called dried plums), but cut them into small pieces. If your child suffers from constipation or just enjoys pureed prunes, you can still use the pureed version as a mix-in. As noted earlier, you can point out to older toddlers that prunes (or dried plums) are like yummy giant raisins. This tends to increase their appeal with the younger set!

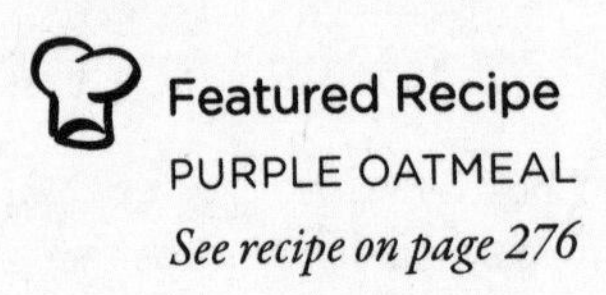

Featured Recipe

PURPLE OATMEAL

See recipe on page 276

3 Avocados

Age: One and two years

PORTION SIZE: 2 tablespoons, one to three times per week

HOW TO SERVE: Diced, sliced, and mashed avocado are all nutritious options. Mashed avocado is a healthy and less spicy alternative to guacamole for toddlers, tasty plain or in a sandwich or burrito. Mashed avocado on bread can also be used instead of mayonnaise. What could be healthier than that?

4 Fish

Age: One and two years

PORTION SIZE: 1 ounce, one to three times per week

HOW TO SERVE: Always cook fish thoroughly, in whatever form or style you prefer. Let your toddler eat a piece of mashed fish off your plate. She can try shellfish too—a tiny bit of shrimp or crab, perhaps? You can experiment with salmon, orange roughy, tilapia, and more, but avoid high-mercury fish such as swordfish and shark (see Safety Tip on fish and mercury on page 33).

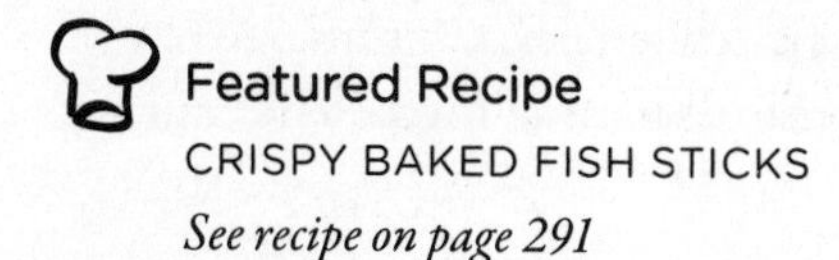

Featured Recipe

CRISPY BAKED FISH STICKS

See recipe on page 291

Safety Tip

Fish and Mercury: Fish is part of a healthy, nutrient-rich diet. That said, due to pollution, fish today contains a form of mercury (methylmercury) which, at certain levels, can affect a young child's developing brain and nervous system.

Recommendations for children:

- Do *not* eat the following, due to extremely high mercury content: shark, king mackerel, swordfish, and tilefish
- Eat no more than two to three child-size portions a week: salmon, tilapia, catfish, trout, pollock, canned light tuna, scallops, crab, and shrimp (less than 6 ounces a week).

5 Yogurt, Cheese, and Milk

Age: One and two years

PORTION SIZE: Three child-size servings a day of dairy products, as follows:

Yogurt: 4 ounces

Cheese: 1 ounce

Milk: 4 to 6 ounces

HOW TO SERVE:

Yogurt: Let your child self-feed with a spoon, helping only as needed. Keep plain Greek or regular yogurt on hand to use in smoothies, along with fresh or frozen berries. Continue to buy full-fat or reduced-fat yogurt with all-natural ingredients and less sugar at this age.

Cheese: Offer diced cheese, string cheese, or cheese slices.

Milk: Offer whole or reduced-fat milk (2 percent) after one year of age. If you are still breast-feeding your baby, continue, but occasionally offer your child sips of regular milk in a cup to get her used to the taste.

For non-breast-feeding infants, offer 16 to 20 ounces a day of whole or reduced-fat milk. Previously it was believed that all toddlers needed whole milk for proper brain development, due to the benefits of dairy fat. Research now shows that reduced fat (2 percent) milk has enough of the needed fat. In addition, 2 percent milk has the same amount of other important nutrients that growing toddlers need. If you have any questions, discuss milk choices with your pediatrician.

Featured Recipe

STOVETOP MACARONI AND CHEESE

See recipe on page 286

➢ Dr. Tanya's Tip: Time for Milk?

For kids over one year of age, milk is the *best* source of vitamin D. (See page 6 for why vitamin D is so important.) After one year of age, whole or 2 percent milk is an important source of nutrition. After age two, nonfat or low-fat milk is best, since those options offer the same nutrition, but with less fat.

➢ Dr. Tanya's Tip: Still Breast-feeding Your Baby?

If you're still breast-feeding your baby after she turns one year of age, good job! You can continue nursing as long as you both desire, but consider offering occasional sips of cold whole or 2 percent milk in a cup to get your toddler used to the taste and temperature. It will make the transition to regular milk easier whenever you decide to wean.

6 Nuts and Nut Butters

Age: One and two years

PORTION SIZE: 1 to 2 teaspoons, two to three times per week

HOW TO SERVE: Kids love peanut butter sandwiches. Try creamy almond butter or peanut butter on whole-grain bread. Nut butter doesn't need to be refrigerated and travels well. It's best to skip the jelly, though; try to get your child used to the taste of only nut butter on whole-grain bread. If you do use jelly, choose one with only natural ingredients—no fake colors or added sugar. Better yet, try mashing your own fruit, perhaps banana or strawberries, to add to a sandwich, or add a touch of honey. Cut any sandwich into quarters and offer one quarter at a time. A typical serving is two quarters (or half a sandwich), but keep leftovers for snacktime. If you make fruit smoothies at home, try adding a teaspoon of nut butter for added protein and fiber.

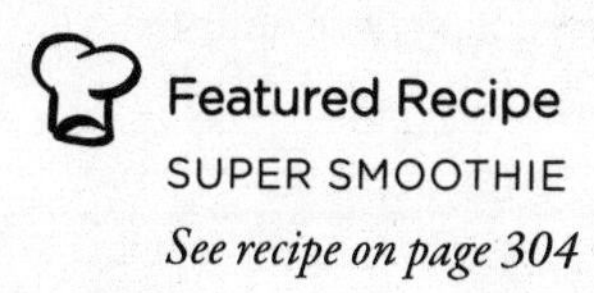

Featured Recipe

SUPER SMOOTHIE

See recipe on page 304

BETH'S GROCERY GUIDE

Which Nut Butter Is Best?

I recommend buying "natural" nut butters—that is, those with no sugar, hydrogenated oil, or preservatives added. Whatever you choose, the main ingredient should definitely be nuts. Natural nut butters tend to separate at room temperature because they don't have extra ingredients and the nut oil naturally rises to the top. You can now find no-stir varieties of natural peanut butter that contain a small amount of palm oil to prevent separation.

Brand A: Natural creamy peanut butter—contains dry-roasted peanuts with or without salt

Brand B: Regular creamy peanut butter—contains roasted peanuts, sugar, hydrogenated vegetable oils, salt

Brand A is the better choice because there's no added sugar or oil. There's no need to buy low-fat peanut butter, however, because the fat in nut butter is a healthy, good-for-you type of fat.

7 Chicken and/or Beans/Lentils

Age: One and two years

PORTION SIZE: 1 to 2 ounces, three to five times per week

HOW TO SERVE: Grilled, baked, broiled, barbecued, poached, sautéed—any way you cook chicken, you can then cut it up into small pieces or tiny strips and serve it to your child plain. Try making a variety of recipes using beans, experimenting to see what your child enjoys. One popular option is a quesadilla, made with mashed beans and shredded cheese heated between two tortillas.

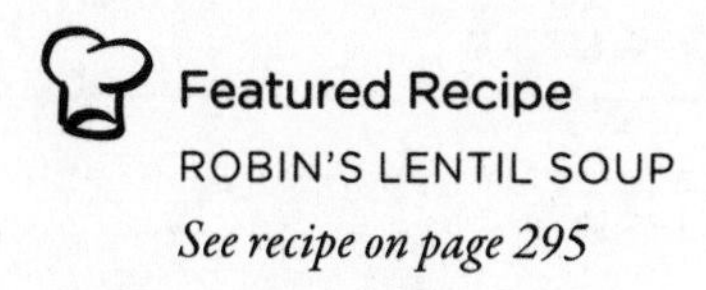

Featured Recipe

ROBIN'S LENTIL SOUP

See recipe on page 295

Kids in the Kitchen

My mom used to buy different varieties of canned beans and use the contents to play counting games with my kids, letting them taste-test the different shapes and colors. Kids can even smash the beans as they count them, if they like.

8 Summer Berries / Winter Citrus

Age: One and two years

PORTION SIZE: ¼ cup, two to three times per week (*Note:* Your toddler should eat *some* type of fruit daily.)

HOW TO SERVE: Offer whole or cut-up berries for snack, as a side to a meal, or as dessert. Berries with yogurt is a popular, healthy dessert choice for toddlers. Not that I recommend lying to toddlers, but some parents call that concoction "ice cream"!

Featured Recipe

BERRY SNACK BARS

See recipe on page 302

9 Green Vegetables

Age: One and two years

PORTION SIZE: ¼ cup, three to five times per week (*Note:* Your toddler should eat *some* type of veggie daily.)

Vegetables

My mantra on produce is "All fruits, all vegetables, all forms." Any dish with at least one ingredient from the produce section is a good choice, so experiment and see what works. Let the kids pick different veggies to buy at the store, even if they don't want to *eat* them initially.

Family-Friendly Vegetable Ideas: Try the vegetable ideas below for the whole family; then modify for your toddler by cutting the cooked veggies into tiny pieces. In addition, your older toddler may like to dip his veggies into anything he wants—Greek yogurt, salad dressing, or melted cheese are three options.

- **Cauliflower:** roast, steam, or serve raw
- **Carrots:** roast or steam
- **Cucumbers (kids tend to enjoy the small, crunchy, seedless Persian variety):** slice on the diagonal for a pretty presentation
- **Bell peppers:** serve slices raw or cut chunks to use in cooking
- **Green beans:** steam and cut into small, bite-size pieces or leave whole for small hands to hold and take bites
- **Edamame:** buy shelled, cooked edamame for convenience
- **Squash:** puree butternut squash; bake spaghetti squash with marinara and cheese
- **Leeks:** use in soups
- **Brussels sprouts:** roast with olive oil, salt, and pepper, then sprinkle with balsamic glaze
- **Asparagus:** steam or roast and serve as "trees"
- **Peas:** steam and serve
- **Sugar snap peas:** serve raw or lightly steam, then toss with butter, salt, and lemon
- **Sweet potatoes:** roast, steam, or mash
- **Corn:** steam and serve either on the cob or off
- **Potatoes:** roast, steam, or mash

HOW TO SERVE: Offer cooked vegetables, since raw may still be too firm at this age, but make the pieces a bit larger than those you served your infant. Try steaming zucchini, which cooks up nice and soft, or bunches of broccoli. Instead of cutting the cooked broccoli into bite-size pieces, let your toddler hold an entire "tree" and take bites. Green beans are usually a child favorite.

Featured Recipe

SAUTÉED GREEN BEANS (OR OTHER VEGGIES)

See recipe on page 294

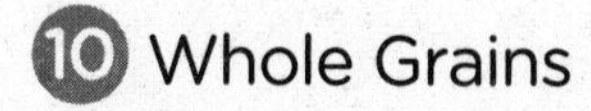

10 Whole Grains

Age: One and two years

PORTION SIZE: ¼ to ½ slice bread, ¼ cup pasta or rice or cereal, daily

HOW TO SERVE: Now is the time many toddlers go "carb crazy." As often as you possibly can, buy the whole-grain version of breads and other grain products to get your kids used to the flavor and texture. It will pay off in the long run. One- to two-year-old children generally enjoy strips of whole-grain bread or toast, as well as whole-grain tortillas, crackers, pasta, waffles, pancakes, and dry cereal.

Featured Recipe

FABULOUS FRENCH TOAST

See recipe on page 278

BETH'S GROCERY GUIDE

Bread

Look for *short* ingredient lists when it comes to bread, crackers, cereal, and other grain-based products. Repeat this mantra as you shop: "Five or less is best; more than ten, think again." Pass on "whole-grain white" products, most of which have fake added fiber and very long ingredient lists.

For truly delicious, healthy bread you can proudly serve, look beyond the grocery store and head to a bakery. The difference is amazing! Choose bread made from 100 percent stone-ground whole wheat, which means the entire grain is left intact until it's ground. In contrast, commercial milling companies remove the bran and germ (the healthiest parts of the wheat kernel) because the extra fat and fiber do not work well with roller mills or mass production. Most "whole-wheat" bread is really white bread with the wheat bran and germ later added back into the recipe.

Fresh bakery bread has fewer of the artificial ingredients—preservatives and dough stabilizers, for example—that are required for a long shelf life, so after a few days you may want to put the loaf in the freezer and take slices out as needed. All the ingredients in a loaf of bread should sound like things you would have in your own kitchen.

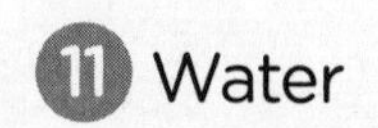

11 Water

Age: One and two years

PORTION SIZE: 2 to 4 ounces, or more as desired, daily

HOW TO SERVE: Offer your child her favorite straw or sippy cup, but also let her practice drinking from a real (open) cup. Getting your toddler used to drinking plain water is the start of a very important lifelong healthy habit.

➢ Dr. Tanya's Tip: Drink Water!

Most people, adults and children alike, should be drinking primarily water. Your child's beverages should be limited to breast milk, milk, and water. No need to start offering juice to your infants or toddlers. (For more information on juice, see chapter 9.) If you're joining the program when your little one is already a toddler, and you haven't yet introduced water to him, now is the time to get him drinking it every day. Whether out of his favorite cup or sports bottle, water should be an ever-present beverage in your house and on the go. As noted in the previous chapter, toddlers who drink water become school-age children who like water and later adults who drink plain water—a super-healthy lifelong habit.

Preschooler Program: Ages Three to Five

If you were brave enough to take your toddler to a restaurant, you probably ate from paper place mats, not proper tablecloths. Cute little toddlers are notoriously messy, rebellious, and constantly on the move. Shortly after entering any restaurant with her two-year-old, Beth (my dietitian and chef) would pick up the food that her toddler had immediately chucked to the ground, and then spend the rest of her time entertaining the toddler outside while other members of her family enjoyed their dinner. Preschoolers are paradise compared to those turbulent toddlers!

The preschool age is a real turning point for feeding and eating. Your three- to five-year-old can more easily express himself, reducing frustration for everyone at the table. He will love my interactive Kids in the Kitchen ideas, presented throughout this section, which involve counting ingredients and even helping to prep, measure, and pour as you cook different recipes. He will feel important as he helps plan a menu and pick food of varying colors at the grocery store.

Here I reveal my Preschooler Program for the Eleven Foundation Foods, specifically tailoring each food for your youngster's growing abilities and independent nature. In chapter 6, we'll delve more deeply into the Preschooler Program and discuss how to get your child to settle in to a more regular eating schedule, enjoy nutrient-rich meals and snacks, become involved in mealtimes, and start to make healthy choices.

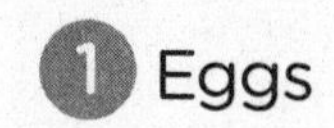

Eggs

Age: Three to five years

PORTION SIZE: 1 egg, two to four times per week

HOW TO SERVE: In addition to the toddler options mentioned earlier, such as scrambled egg, omelet, frittata, or French toast, try making an egg sandwich using whole-grain bread/toast or a hollowed-out bagel. Just place the scrambled egg on the bread or inside the bagel and serve! Another option is making a healthy egg-salad sandwich, a protein-rich vegetarian option for lunch. If you make French toast, it's still best to avoid syrup and other sweet toppings; do so for as long as possible. Kids who don't grow up with syrup, sugar, or whipped cream on their French toast don't choose it on their own when they're older.

Featured Recipe

MAKE-AHEAD BREAKFAST BURRITOS

See recipe on page 277

Family Feeding

The whole family can enjoy egg dishes like French toast. A weekend breakfast may be more relaxing than dinnertime, and you can now try more adventurous breakfast dishes along with family favorites. Just avoid serving a young child anything undercooked.

Kids in the Kitchen

Let your child count the eggs as you crack them into the bowl. She can also help you whisk the eggs and dunk the bread into the French toast mixture.

2 Prunes

Age: Three to five years

PORTION SIZE: 1 to 2 prunes, two to three times per week, or daily if needed

HOW TO SERVE: One prune daily is great for a snack. Look for prunes sold in cute little single-serve packages so fingers won't get sticky. School-age kids can simply tear open the wrapper and pop the fruit into their mouth . . . yum. Just to be safe, so they don't choke, cut the prunes in half for three- or four-year-olds. If your child is constipated, up the amount to two or three prunes. As noted earlier, I often use prunes to treat (and especially prevent) constipation. I recommend one to four prunes, depending on the severity of the constipation. Definitely try prunes before you try a stool softener. They are natural, healthy, and much gentler on a child's system.

Featured Recipe

PERSONALIZED TRAIL MIX

See recipe on page 305

3 Avocados

Age: Three to five years

PORTION SIZE: 2 to 3 tablespoons or more as desired, one to two times per week

HOW TO SERVE: Continue to offer avocado any way your preschooler enjoys it, including sliced, mashed, in chunks, or as part of guacamole.

Featured Recipe

TURKEY AVOCADO WRAP

See recipe on page 290

Kids in the Kitchen

Preschoolers love a tactile experience. Give your preschooler a spoon to scrape out the insides of an avocado. He can use a potato masher or fork to mash the pulp, and then spread it himself on a tortilla or slice of bread.

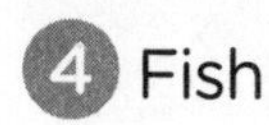

4 Fish

Age: Three to five years

PORTION SIZE: 1 to 2 ounces, one to three times per week

HOW TO SERVE: Sandwiches are a great way to get more fish into your preschooler's diet. Start offering tuna and salmon sandwiches at this age. See the earlier Safety Tip on fish and mercury (p. 33) for lower-mercury fish options and recommended amounts. My boys like their tuna sandwiches made with a little bit of mayonnaise and some finely chopped celery.

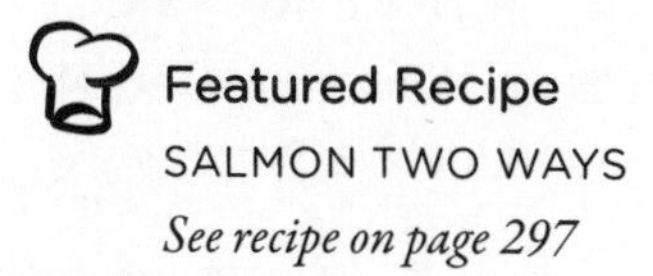

Featured Recipe

SALMON TWO WAYS

See recipe on page 297

Safety Tip

The Truth About Tuna: Albacore tuna, both canned and fresh, has approximately a three times higher methylmercury concentration than canned light tuna. Several brands of albacore and light tuna are now available that contain line-caught fish, smaller and naturally lower in mercury.

BETH'S GROCERY GUIDE

Fish Sticks

Store-bought fish sticks are often used as a convenient, kid-friendly food for lunch or dinner. This is okay once in a while, but avoid serving store-bought fish sticks every day. They aren't really a good alternative to a piece of fresh fish, because they're not as nutritious and they don't help your child get used to the appearance, taste, and smell of regular fish. If you do buy fish sticks, read the ingredient lists and choose a brand that names only short, recognizable ingredients.

See our recipe for Crispy Baked Fish Sticks on page 291. It offers an easy way to make your own healthy, tasty fish sticks.

Family Feeding

Serve fish to the entire family if you want your child to like fish. Offer fish at least once a week for dinner. Fish takes on so many different flavors, depending on your preparation: you can marinate it or put it in any sauce you like. Don't be afraid to add some seasoning and fat (olive oil, canola oil, or a little butter) to your fish.

5 Yogurt, Cheese, and Milk

Age: Three to five years

PORTION SIZE: Three child-size servings a day of dairy products, as follows:

Milk: 4 to 6 ounces

Yogurt: 4 ounces

Cheese: 1 ounce

HOW TO SERVE:

Milk: If your child has been eating yogurt since around six months of age and drinking milk since one year, it should be easy to continue offering dairy products three times a day as recommended; this enables your child to get enough of the nine essential nutrients provided in milk and other dairy products.

If you're joining the program when your child is already a preschooler and isn't yet accustomed to dairy products, if your child has gone on a temporary milk strike, or if your child simply refuses to drink milk (as some do), other options to ensure three servings of dairy a day include offering milk with cereal, adding milk or yogurt to smoothies, and including yogurt and cheese as part of meals and snacks.

Family Feeding

All members of the family can now enjoy any of the following together: a smoothie made with yogurt, cereal with milk, a bagel with cream cheese, a bean and cheese burrito, or a yogurt parfait. It is much easier to make the same meal for everyone, adapting it slightly for different tastes or abilities, than it is to make separate meals.

Yogurt: Many preschoolers are away from home over the lunch hour. If that's the case in your household, the best way to ensure that your child is getting three servings of dairy daily is to include one in the lunchbox. Send yogurt in your child's lunch with an ice pack to keep it cool. You can also buy yogurt tubes and stick them in the freezer. Pack one in the morning, and it will thaw by lunchtime.

Yogurt is a great snack food too. Continue to buy plain yogurt and add berries and honey for extra flavor, or use yogurt as a base for fruit smoothies or for dipping. Make yogurt a meal by adding whole-grain cereal and berries. Please resist the urge to buy yogurt with cookie or sugared-cereal toppings. If yogurt has such toppings, it is *dessert,* not healthy yogurt! Likewise, yogurt should not contain any fake colors.

Cheese: String cheese is another great lunch option. One of Beth's daughters likes her string cheese already "in strings," which is very easy to accommodate—Beth just sends it in a small reusable container.

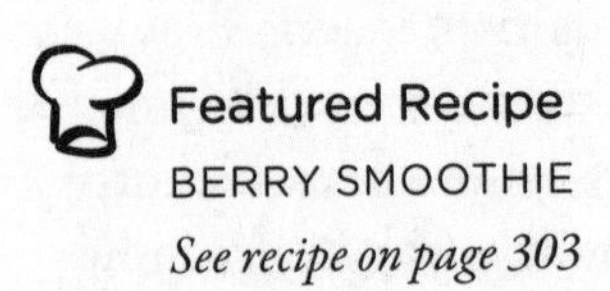

Featured Recipe

BERRY SMOOTHIE

See recipe on page 303

Kids in the Kitchen

Bananas dipped in vanilla yogurt taste like marshmallows. Apple slices or pretzels dipped in yogurt are also yummy. Give your kids the ingredients and let them dip away! If your preschooler likes store-bought yogurt drinks, put them on a low shelf in the refrigerator with straws nearby. Beth's older daughter insisted that her bendy straw go upside-down into the yogurt drink—for years!

➢ Dr. Tanya's Tip: Flavored Milks

I prefer that all kids drink plain milk, but if your child likes flavored milk—especially at school, at a party, or for an after-sports treat—it's a great option to deliver protein, calcium, vitamin D, and the other essential nutrients in milk.

Research has shown that chocolate milk is a great option for after-sports snacks. It has delicious taste, with just the right amount of carbs, protein, and other nutrients to help your child (and professional athletes) replenish their energy stores.

Some parents are concerned about the amount of added sugar in chocolate milk. Let's talk about it. One brand of low-fat chocolate milk has 26 grams of sugar per cup. Given that low-fat plain milk has 13 grams of naturally occurring sugar per cup, we're talking about 13 grams of *added* sugar. One popular juice pouch contains 13 to 16 grams of added sugar per cup, while a popular sports drink has 14 grams of added sugar per cup—but neither of these products has any of the nutrition found in milk. Studies show that children who drink flavored milk do not consume more added sugar in their diets, but they do drink more milk overall and thus meet more of their nutrient needs.[4]

You can make your own chocolate milk using a small amount of organic chocolate syrup. Overall, though, Beth and I both believe that low-fat chocolate milk is a good alternative to juice or sports drinks.

BETH'S GROCERY GUIDE

Brand Loyalty

Kids start developing strong brand loyalty by preschool age—and sometimes even as toddlers. In families that have not followed my program from the beginning, I constantly hear parents in my office explain, "Jake will eat only the cookie yogurt, or the cereal with the bunny on the box." My answer: "Then stop buying it for him."

I know it's difficult. You worry that your child will refuse healthier brands—or refuse to eat, period. Don't worry: he will not go hungry! You don't want to start the vicious cycle of buying *only* the brands your child prefers. It's fine to indulge a few favorite brands and types of foods—especially healthy foods—up to a certain point. We all have preferences about what types of foods we like and how we want them prepared. But draw the line at buying junk foods your child insists upon—save them for occasional treats only.

6 Nuts and Nut Butters

Age: Three to five years

PORTION SIZE: 1 tablespoon nut butter, or 3 to 6 whole nuts cut up, two to four times per week

HOW TO SERVE: Nuts are portable protein! They offer a fun way to get heart-healthy fats and fiber as well. You can now start giving whole/slivered/crushed nuts if your child is developmentally ready. When offering a small nut (such as a peanut), give only one nut at a time. Crush or break bigger nuts into smaller pieces. Offer any nuts in any form, but as always, keep a close eye on your child and make sure that she is eating only one at a time and chewing thoroughly, to prevent choking. Nut butters are also wonderful spread on apple chunks or added to smoothies. See our Super Smoothie recipe (p. 304) for a yummy nut butter drink.

Featured Recipe

ALMOND-OAT GRANOLA BARS

See recipe on page 301

Safety Tip

Nuts as a Choking Hazard: It's well known that whole nuts are a choking hazard for infants and small children. That said, after your child reaches age three, you can offer him small whole nuts one at a time, watching him carefully. Teach him to fully chew each nut. Don't offer nuts while walking around or while riding in the car (since in a vehicle you can't easily reach him if needed).

Nuts and Trail Mix

Nuts: The best options are unsalted nuts, those made with less salt, or your own combination of salted and unsalted nuts. A store near us sells nuts labeled "50 percent less salt" in individually wrapped snack packs—very yummy! Ingredient lists on nut packaging should be *extremely* short.

Trail Mix: Trail mix is a good way to include more nuts in your child's diet in a fun, portable way. If you buy premade trail mix, be careful: many are loaded with sugar, include *tons* of ingredients, and are about as healthy as a candy bar. One example I've seen is ultra-processed and contains *nine* different sources of sugar—and it's marketed as a healthy, nutritious, high-energy snack!

A better alternative is to make your own trail mix with nuts, raisins (or other dried fruit pieces), a few pretzels, and maybe some whole-grain cereal or chocolate or yogurt chips—all much better for you than any trail mix you can buy at the store. Let your kids help by choosing their favorite items to go with the nuts of their choice.

Safety Tip

Nuts in Schools: More and more preschool and elementary schools are either completely nut-free, have peanut-free zones, or have nut-free tables. There are many nut butter options besides peanut butter; if your school is only peanut-free, try almond or cashew butter. If your school is completely nut-free, sunflower seed butter and soy-nut butter are both great options. Additional nut-free alternatives are being developed that contain ingredients such as golden peas.

7 Chicken and/or Beans/Lentils

Age: Three to five years

PORTION SIZE: 2 ounces, three to five times per week

HOW TO SERVE: Continue to make and serve your child chicken in many forms—grilled, baked, barbecued, sautéed—basically, any way that you'd eat it yourself. You may discover a certain preparation or sauce that your child particularly likes. My boys love the grilled organic chicken breasts that my husband cooks on the barbecue. They are eager to try *whatever* they see Daddy cooking in the backyard!

Avoid processed frozen breaded chicken pieces whenever possible, whether at home or eating out. If you're at a restaurant, it's generally healthier to order chicken for your kids off the adult menu and cut the food to an appropriate portion size. This is the age, though, when lots of families fight the fast-food battle. Many kids want fried chicken tenders, and many parents give in because it's easy and avoids a conflict. Remember that fried foods should be "once in a while" foods—not daily forms of protein.

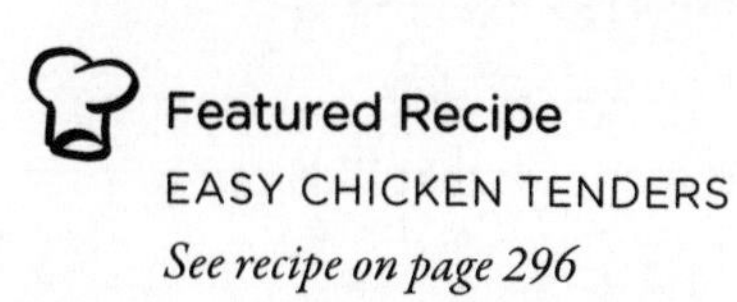

Featured Recipe

EASY CHICKEN TENDERS

See recipe on page 296

Family Feeding

For a vegetarian alternative or to add variety to your child's protein intake, introduce beans early and frequently. Remember, they are high in fiber, protein, vitamins, and minerals. All forms are great—canned or dry, or even vegetarian refried. Offer beans alone, as well as mashed in a quesadilla or with a potato. Add them to your (adult) salad. If you don't eat beans, chances are your kids won't either.

Kids in the Kitchen

Let your child help bread chicken—she can whisk the eggs, dust the chicken pieces in flour, and even coat them with bread crumbs.

Safety Tip

Raw Chicken: Be very careful when handling raw chicken. Make sure you use a separate cutting board, wash any knives and surfaces well after contact, discard any marinade that had contact with raw poultry, and of course wash your hands well and teach your kids to wash their hands well (that is, with warm soapy water for twenty seconds) after handling. Cook poultry to a safe minimum internal temperature of 165°F.

8 Summer Berries / Winter Citrus

Age: Three to five years

PORTION SIZE: ¼ to ½ cup, two to three times per week (*Note:* Your preschooler should eat *some* type of fruit daily.)

HOW TO SERVE: Keep washed berries in easy-to-grab containers in the refrigerator. They're a nutritious, easy snack that kids can help themselves to any time of day.

Blend fresh or frozen berries into smoothies for an afternoon snack or dessert.

For citrus in winter, clementines are a perfect lunchbox fruit or after-school snack.

Featured Recipe

WHOLE-WHEAT BURSTING-WITH-BLUEBERRY MUFFINS

See recipe on page 281

Kids in the Kitchen

Use berries to teach colors and counting. Preschoolers love to eat things they can count! They also enjoy lining up berries by color, or making a smiley face using orange segments.

Family Feeding

Make a healthy smoothie with your kids. Let them count and throw in whatever berries or citrus fruits they choose. Alternatively, a layered parfait of yogurt, granola, and berries is a delicious snack or dessert that kids and adults alike can enjoy.

Green Vegetables

Age: Three to five years

PORTION SIZE: ¼ to ½ cup, three to five times per week (*Note:* Your child should eat *some* type of veggie daily.)

HOW TO SERVE: Serve veggies—alternating green with other colors—with lunch, with dinner, and as one snack a day. For your green veggies, try cold cut-up cucumbers or snap peas with lunch or as an after-school snack and hot broccoli, zucchini, or asparagus with dinner. As suggested earlier, make your kids broccoli "trees" to gain their interest (and feel free to offer dips like marinara, ranch dressing, or cheese). Let your kids help plan meals, choose veggies to buy at the store, and help cook at least one meal a week. Use a rainbow chart to get your children excited about trying new vegetables in different colors.

Featured Recipe

SUPER-QUICK DECONSTRUCTED SALAD BAR

See recipe on page 288

Cooking Help Desk

Doctoring Veggies: Cook vegetables for your preschooler just as you would for the rest of the family. If your child doesn't love a plain preparation, try sprinkling cheese on top or letting him dip veggies in his favorite sauce (e.g., ranch dressing, hummus, barbecue sauce, or ketchup).

Family Feeding

At least once a week involve your children in cooking a meal. This is a great way to teach them about nutritious eating and helping out at home. If you try a new recipe together, let your kids introduce the new dish to the family. A child could even name it after herself—for example, Zoey's Veggie Lasagna.

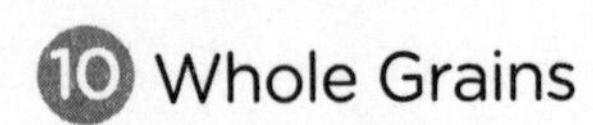

10 Whole Grains

Age: Three to five years

PORTION SIZE: ½ to 1 slice whole-grain bread, ¼ to ½ cup pasta/rice/cereal, ½ to 1 whole-grain tortilla daily

HOW TO SERVE: When you think about what grain products to serve your preschooler, stick to options with a short ingredient list and at least 3 grams of fiber per serving, without fake colors, and most of your choices will be good. Try making a wrap—put the protein and/or veggie in a tortilla, wrap tightly, then cut diagonally to make pretty little slices that show what's inside.

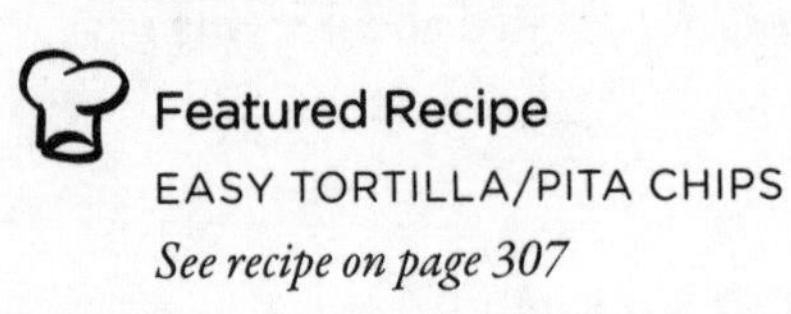

Featured Recipe

EASY TORTILLA/PITA CHIPS

See recipe on page 307

Safety Tip

Popcorn: Popcorn, if not topped with too many extras, is a great high-fiber snack most kids love. Air-popped is healthiest. After age three is a good time to introduce popcorn, but watch your child carefully while she's eating it. Popcorn is a potential choking hazard and best to avoid before that age.

Cooking Help Desk

Whole-Grain Breakfast Ideas: For an easy and quick breakfast, try whole-grain cereal (dry or with milk), a piece of whole-grain toast, oatmeal, or a whole-grain waffle. You can also make French toast with 100 percent whole-wheat bread, and save extra in the fridge for a couple days' worth of breakfast.

One of Beth's daughters likes to have matzo brei (an egg dish that uses matzo) in the mornings—so Beth makes a big batch and uses half regular matzo and half whole-wheat matzo.

Kids in the Kitchen

Let your preschooler stir her own oatmeal and add her toppings, such as raisins, cranberries, or a touch of honey. My kids even put dry whole-grain cereal on top of their oatmeal. If you're the adventurous type, or have a dog (for easy cleanup), let your child pour her own cereal into a bowl.

11 Water

Age: Three to five years

PORTION SIZE: 2 to 4 ounces, or more as desired, daily

HOW TO SERVE: If your child goes to preschool, invest in an insulated cup he can take to school daily. Metal Thermos-type cups stay cool throughout the day. Packing water instead of a juice box will get your child used to drinking plain water instead of sweet-tasting beverages. I promise you will thank me years later, when your child loves to drink plain water and voluntarily passes on juices and sodas!

Kids in the Kitchen

Start letting your child be responsible for getting his own drink at meals, especially dinnertime. Store your child's cups (and other dishes too at this age) where he can reach them, and make it easy for him to get water on his own throughout the day.

PART TWO

Feeding Your Baby and Toddler

3.

Milk Matters

From Breast to Bean and Every Milk in Between

Let's start with the basics. Before you jump into the Eleven Foundation Foods with your infant, you'll be offering an even more foundational food. We all know that a baby's healthy diet starts with milk—specifically, breast milk, which is the most nutritious first milk for any infant. It will prime your baby's brain, digestive tract, immune system, and palate for a healthy life. It's through breast milk that your baby will get a first taste of nutrients and flavors from your diet, setting her on a path to lifelong healthy eating and nutrition.

Breast-feeding: Your Breasts Know Best

As I write this chapter, I have a one-month-old (my third son) attached to my breast. I breast-fed my first two boys too, and each time it was a unique and special experience. It's only natural that the first food you feed your child will be your breast milk. Breast milk is nature's perfect superfood, providing all the protein, sugar, fat, and calories your baby needs to grow and develop. It also contains ingredients to help your baby stay healthy, including antibodies, immune factors, enzymes, and white blood cells.

These nutrients help protect your baby against diseases and infections not only while she's breast-feeding, but in many cases for life. Breast-fed babies have fewer ear, respiratory tract, and diarrheal infections. They are also at lower risk for many childhood diseases, such as asthma, diabetes, and obesity. And breast-feeding is not just good for babies; it has many documented benefits for mothers too, including a decreased future risk of cancer and diabetes and a faster return to prepregnancy weight. Every time I nurse I think to myself: breast-feeding burns three to five hundred calories a day—the equivalent of a three-mile run!

Although breast-feeding is natural, most babies aren't born experts (and neither are we moms!). It may take days (or even weeks) for you and your little one to catch on, especially if your milk supply is a little

➢ Dr. Tanya's Tip: Vitamin D

The American Academy of Pediatrics recommends that all breast-fed infants receive 400 IU of vitamin D daily, starting within the first week of life. Breast milk generally does not contain enough vitamin D, which is important to prevent illness and build strong bones. Luckily, there are many good-tasting liquid vitamin D supplements available for infants. I suggest putting the dose directly on your breast or squirting it into your infant's mouth during a feed. As always, follow the dosing directions on the vitamin supplement you are giving your baby and store it out of a child's reach.

slow to come in. Try not to get discouraged. Don't be afraid to ask for help from day one, if not before. Breast-feeding takes patience and can be hard work initially, but keep at it because the benefits for your baby's health as well as your own are immense.

So how long should you breast-feed? Ideally, for at least your baby's first year of life, but continue breast-feeding for as long as you and your baby desire. Any amount of breast milk you provide your baby is beneficial.

Note the following recommendation from a policy statement issued by the American Academy of Pediatrics (AAP):

> *The AAP recommends exclusive breastfeeding for about 6 months, with continuation of breastfeeding for 1 year or longer as mutually desired by mother and infant, a recommendation concurred to by the WHO [World Health Organization] and the Institute of Medicine.*[5]

Mom's Diet During Breast-feeding

Don't diet after your baby's birth! You are a human feeding factory working overtime—especially for the first six months. You need to consume three to five hundred extra calories daily to fuel your milk production. I enjoyed the excuse to eat a variety of tasty, healthy foods, and with every bite I knew that what I was eating and drinking was passing through my body and breast milk to my boys. This is your baby's first taste of flavorful nutrition. The more you expose your body and your baby to a variety of the Eleven Foundation Foods, the healthier you and your baby will be for life. The best advice I received about nutrition while breast-feeding came from a lactation educator and baby nurse friend of mine, Polly. She said, "Eat more healthy carbs—oatmeal every day and whole grains at every meal and snack—to increase breast milk production." Boy, did that work! In addition, it's very important to stay well hydrated with a combination of water, decaffeinated tea/coffee, diluted juice, milk, fruits, vegetables, soups, and salads.

Bottom line: if you want to lose baby weight, cutting out junk food and sugar is fine—eating healthily is *always* a good idea—but don't cut calories too drastically, especially in the form of whole-grain carbs.

Sometimes a nursing mother will need to eliminate a certain food from her diet because it causes a problem for the breast-feeding infant. If you notice signs of an allergy (such as a rash or wheezing) or signs of a sensitivity (such as fussiness or blood in the stool), call your pediatrician right away. Dairy products, such as cow's milk, are the most common offenders. In some cases, an infant may develop blood in the stool, which can be due to sensitivity to dairy in mom's diet. In such instances, a mom may need to eliminate dairy products temporarily from her diet. The good news is most babies will outgrow this reaction by one to two years of age. Ask your pediatrician if you're concerned that your baby may have an allergy or a sensitivity to a food in your diet.

I found that when I ate certain foods, especially in excess amounts—foods such as broccoli, beans, and lentils—my nursing baby would be a bit more gassy and fussy. I learned the hard way when Beth delivered me an absolutely delicious quinoa and broccoli casserole. I indulged too much, and my son was up crying and gassy all night. Although I've seen no research to prove this, my baby nurse–friend Polly says that in her experience, the foods most likely to make babies gassy are broccoli, cauliflower, cabbage, beans, and lentils. I have to say that, based on my personal experience as a mom and a pediatrician, I do agree!

Physical Activity While Nursing

As soon as your ob-gyn gives you the green light, rely on exercise to help you stay healthy and get back to your prepregnancy shape. My jogging stroller was my savior when my oldest son was born: every morning, no matter how tired I was, I put my son in the stroller and went for a walk (to my favorite coffee shop and back).

Weather not cooperating? There are plenty of indoor exercises you can do with your baby, or while your baby is napping, to help burn calories, tone your body, and get back into shape.

Donor Breast Milk

We've established the benefits of breast milk, but there are women who for a variety of reasons are not able to provide their baby with their own breast milk. Good news: there are human milk banks that screen milk donors and safely collect, process, test, and store donor breast milk. This is a great option for adopted infants and infants born through surrogacy or other instances where the mother is not able to nurse. Some hospitals now provide donor breast milk for premature babies or babies with special health issues.

The Human Milk Banking Association of North America (www.hmbana.org) is a good resource for more information on donor breast milk.

Infant Formula

While breast milk is the best source of nutrition for your newborn, if you aren't able to breast-feed, choose not to, or would like to occasionally supplement, talk to your pediatrician about alternatives. In such cases there are many commercial infant formula options available that are specially made to support a baby's growth and development. Infant formula has come a long way, and recent additions to infant formula (such as probiotics, prebiotics, lutein, and the fatty acids DHA and ARA) really provide babies with all the nutrients they need to grow and thrive. If you are feeding your infant formula, simply substitute formula for breast milk in our feeding charts, advice, and recipes. Yes, your formula-fed baby can still go to Harvard!

The one thing I strongly advise *against* is homemade infant formula. I've never met a parent who didn't want the best for his or her infant, and

> **➢ Dr. Tanya's Tip: Mommy Guilt**
>
> **I'd like to take a moment to talk about Mommy Guilt. We all have it at one time or another. Whether Mommy Guilt is due to feeding your baby formula or going back to work (those are often the top two of a long list of many), we all need to understand that it's part of being a mom and being human. You will face many decisions as a parent, and what's most important is that you choose what's best for your family and for you as a person (not what *other* people think is best). That way you can be happy, stay healthy, and enjoy being there for your child.**

certainly good intentions lie behind homemade formula: some parents feel that making their own infant formula is "healthier" or "more natural" than buying commercial infant formula. It's important to know that giving a baby homemade infant formula can lead to potentially serious health consequences as well as poor growth and development. Among the health hazards, some homemade infant formulas contain raw animal milk, which can lead to serious and deadly infections. If you choose to use infant formula, please buy one that is commercially available in the United States, which means that it meets the FDA standards for nutrition and safety as set by the Infant Formula Act, which was developed to safeguard the nutritional health of all infants.

Spit-Up and Reflux

As a pediatrician, I couldn't write a book about feeding babies without addressing spit-up. Although babies spit up for various reasons, by far the most common is reflux. *Reflux* is the term for stomach contents going the wrong way out of the stomach—that is, going back up into the mouth, instead of down and into the intestines. Essentially all babies reflux, at least a little, because they spend so much time on their back, without the help of gravity to move their food down. In addition, in babies the esophagus—the feeding tube—is short, and the muscle at the bottom of the feeding tube and the top of the stomach is relaxed and floppy. This allows food in the stomach to more easily come back up and out of the mouth—hence, spit-up!

In addition to spit-up, reflux can sometimes cause other symptoms, such as pain or discomfort. Generally speaking, though, as long as a baby with reflux is eating well, gaining weight normally, and isn't too uncomfortable, no treatment is needed. The feeding tube will lengthen and the muscle will naturally tighten with time, so the reflux usually resolves by about one year of age.

Some infants with reflux will continue to occasionally spit up into toddlerhood if they overeat; occasional throwing up may even last into childhood, especially if kids overeat or eat too much junk. My second son would throw up a few times a year, usually after eating too many crackers at a sporting event or while traveling home from a family event where he ate way too much. This is normal and fine, though it's a reminder to watch out for and regulate how much and what your kids are eating.

Safety Tip

When to Call Your Pediatrician About Spit-Up: Call your pediatrician if your baby spits up frequently (after more than half of his feeds per day) and/or has any of the following:

- Failure to feed well or gain weight appropriately
- Respiratory symptoms such as coughing, wheezing, or choking
- Discomfort after a feed (indicated by crying and/or arching)
- Projectile spit-up (spit-up that shoots out)
- Bloody spit-up

Feeding via Baby Bottle

Even if you're exclusively feeding your baby breast milk, if you plan to return to work or ever want to go out to a dinner and movie without your baby in tow, then you will need to teach your baby to drink from a bottle. Pumping and storing breast milk to be served in a bottle also gives others the opportunity to feed and bond with your baby, while giving you a much-needed break.

The best time to introduce a bottle to your baby is around three or four weeks, once breast-feeding is well established. Once you've gotten your baby to take a bottle, continue to offer her a bottle once a day (at least), so she doesn't forget the process or simply refuse the bottle. Bottles can be used until around twelve to fifteen months of age to provide milk and water for your baby. It's best to avoid putting juice in a bottle, however, for two reasons: it will get your baby used to wanting sweet things, and it's not good for her erupting teeth.

Weaning to a Cup

Good health starts with breast milk whenever possible, as we've seen. But as children get older, they move from breast and/or bottle to cup. It's a good idea to get your child used to drinking from a cup early on. Here's the advice I give parents on how to wean a child to a cup:

Six to Twelve Months

Introduce a sippy or straw cup around six to nine months of age and keep offering it. Don't get discouraged if your infant doesn't accept it immediately. Start with water to avoid messy spills, but as soon as possible, try breast milk in the cup. It may sound strange to put breast milk in a sippy cup, but it's the best way to ensure that your older infant will drink *everything* from a cup. I see too many parents who put milk only in a bottle;

then later, when they get rid of the bottle, their toddler refuses to drink milk. Once your child has mastered drinking milk from a sippy or straw cup, you can begin to wean him off the bottle, with the goal of having the bottle completely gone by twelve to eighteen months of age.

Twelve Months and Up

After age one, the transition from bottle to cup can be more challenging, especially if your toddler has declared his bottle a security or comfort object. You can try weaning him off the bottle gradually, but often after fifteen months of age cold turkey is the way to go. Choose a day, gather up all the bottles, and give them away. If your child is able to understand, you can warn him the day before that you'll be giving the bottles to a baby who needs them (perhaps a cousin or a baby next door). He may cry, scream, and even refuse to drink for a day or two (don't worry, he won't get dehydrated), but he'll quickly forget and soon take to that sippy or straw cup with a cute character on it that you bought just for him.

The Ongoing Importance of Milk

By eighteen months your child should be off the bottle, and by two or three years he should be off the cute sippy cup and drinking from a regular cup (a *cute* regular cup is okay). Straw cups are still useful on the go, however, or for water on the bedroom nightstand, to help decrease spillage.

After switching to a regular cup, your child should still be drinking three child-size servings of milk a day. As you saw in the previous chapter, milk contains nine essential nutrients, including protein, calcium, and vitamin D, making it one of the most nutrient-rich beverages kids can enjoy. Even though your child is now *eating* many of his calories, milk is still an important part of his overall diet.

Even though I recommend that parents give their children cow's milk (or soy milk if they're allergic), there are reasons you might choose a different kind of milk. For example, you might have a family history of dairy allergies or lactose intolerance, you might feel that almond milk is more nutritious, or you or your child might prefer the taste of rice milk. It's important to know, though, that some so-called milks are really more like fortified white juice and contain little protein or nutrients (see Beth's Grocery Guide on page 71).

On the other hand, some toddlers are milkaholics! They would rather guzzle down bottle after bottle of milk than eat real food. While milk is a very nutritious part of your toddler's diet, way too much of a good thing can fill up a tiny belly and not leave room for nutritious, iron-rich foods. Aim for three 6-ounce servings (or 16 to 20 ounces a day, total) from a cup.

Compare Calories

The calorie data in the chart on page 71 ("Milk and Its Alternatives") is based on 8 ounces of beverage. All of the milk alternatives in the chart are available fortified with calcium and vitamins A and D; choose only versions that are.

Starting at age one, toddlers and preschoolers have high calorie needs (approximately 1,000 to 1,400 calories a day, depending on a child's size and activity level), but their total volume of intake is generally low because they fill up so quickly. If you switch your child from cow's milk to almond milk at 16 ounces a day, that leaves a gap of 180 calories you have to make up somewhere else!

Compare Protein

Protein is important for your child to properly gain weight, grow, and develop. You do not need to push a certain number of grams daily, or even count grams, but most young kids need a good source of protein at least three times daily. As you can see from the chart below, if you swap 16 ounces of cow's milk for rice, almond, or coconut milk, that leaves at least a 14-gram protein deficit, which is a lot to make up every day! I've seen a few toddlers having trouble gaining weight because they were

BETH'S GROCERY GUIDE

Milk and Its Alternatives

There are a lot of different milk products in the stores today. Here's everything you need to know about choosing milk and milk alternatives for toddlers and young children.

	Calories	Grams of protein	Notes
Cow's milk	150	8	
Soy milk	110	8	
Goat's milk	142	8	Use only if fortified with folate; check with your pediatrician first
Rice milk	120	1	High in calories, low in protein
Almond milk	30–60*	1	Low in both calories and protein
Coconut milk	45–80*	0	Moderate in calories, low in protein, controversial in fat content
Hemp milk	140	3	Low in protein, not widely available

*Calories vary by brand and if product is sweetened or unsweetened.

drinking almond or coconut milk and lacked other foods to make up the balance of protein. The best milk options with a high protein punch are cow's milk and soy milk. Goat's milk has similar protein compared to cow's milk and soy milk, has fewer nutrients than cow's milk, and is deficient in folate and B_{12}, a deficiency that can lead to anemia.

Look at the Child's Growth

Scenario A

A two-year-old drinks almond milk from a cup (6 ounces twice a day) and is growing well. Her height and weight are stable on the growth chart. She has an egg most mornings, often has yogurt or string cheese as a snack, and eats dinner with her family at night, often consuming chicken, turkey, or fish, or perhaps a bean and rice burrito or lentil soup.

Verdict. No problem. The child's height and weight are good, and she is getting protein from foods as well as milk. No changes are needed.

Scenario B

An eighteen-month-old switched from drinking 24 ounces of cow's milk to 24 ounces of almond milk daily. The child isn't eating much at lunch or dinner but seems to do well at breakfast. He had been gaining steadily along the 25th percentile for weight/age, but since the switch his weight gain has dropped off and he is now at the 10th percentile.

Verdict. The low-calorie, low-protein beverage is filling up the child's tummy but not providing enough nutrients. His parents should change him to a higher-calorie, higher-protein beverage (such as cow's milk), or decrease his bottles and increase quantities of high-protein solid foods such as eggs, chicken, fish, beans, cheese, and nut butters.

Q&A: Solutions for Real Parent Questions

Giving Up Milk Along with the Bottle

Q: I took away the bottle, and now my toddler refuses to drink milk. What should I do?

A: Continue to offer milk and show her that you drink milk, too. You can take a drink and then invite your toddler to join you. Make drinking milk fun. I would say "Cheers!" and clink my cup with my second son's during his milk strike at eighteen months, after we got rid of his beloved bottle. I continued to offer him milk and let him watch his brother and me drinking milk. After trying out a variety of different sippy, straw, and regular cup options, he eventually started to drink milk again.

If your child is off milk completely, you may need to be a bit creative to get the needed calcium and vitamin D into her diet. Children need three servings a day—but remember that these are child-size servings of 4 to 6 ounces (compared to an adult 8-ounce serving). Try milk in cereal, smoothies, and soup, plus cheese and yogurt.

Look at the Child's Diet as a Whole

If your child is eating a great variety of foods, and growing well, there likely won't be any problem if you choose to stop giving cow's milk. If you want to eliminate *all* dairy from your child's diet, however, it is important that you meet with a registered dietitian to make sure the youngster is getting an adequately balanced diet with enough nutrients from other sources.

As you may have realized, I'm a big dairy fan. Milk really is a good source of nine essential nutrients that many kids don't get enough of, including protein, calcium, vitamin D, and potassium. I find that kids who enjoy drinking milk and eating yogurt tend to grow up to be healthier eaters and drinkers overall. Of course, you can still raise a healthy child without dairy, but it's important to remember that not all nondairy milks are created equal and many lack protein and other essential nutrients that growing kids (and adults) need. I still drink my milk every day.

Remember This

- Breast milk is full of nutrients your growing baby needs. I recommend breast-feeding up to one year of age—or longer, as child and mom desire.
- As a rule, choose breast milk over formula. When that's not possible, use commercially available, FDA-approved formula. Stay away from homemade formula, which can be dangerous.
- Cow's milk has strong health benefits for older children. It provides nine important nutrients, including protein, calcium, vitamin D, and healthy calories to help your child grow.
- Get your child used to drinking milk from a cup early on so that it's easier to wean her from the bottle.
- Different types of milk have differing amounts of nutrition. It's important to know exactly what your child is drinking.

4.

The Infant Program

Skip the Baby-Food Aisle and Start Solids the Right Way

As I previewed in chapter 2, there is a specific, easy-to-follow program that I recommend for all of my patients as they are introducing their little ones to solid foods for the first time. Before we get to the specifics of how to use the Eleven Foundation Foods Program to feed your baby, let's take a look at all the options for baby food that exist, and see which is best.

We've been taught, whether by other parents or by advertising, that purchasing baby food is the best, easiest, and perhaps only way to feed our little ones. However, there's a better way to start your baby on solid foods. I tell parents that they should actually skip the baby-food aisle altogether. That's right! Throw out the white baby cereal, get rid of the chicken puree combo that smells like dog food, and liberate yourself from multi-ingredient pouches that contain only miniscule amounts of the healthy ingredients listed on the front. With a few easy steps, you can make your own healthy, tasty, cost-effective food for your baby.

Before you toss this book in disbelief or disgust, let's examine the benefits and drawbacks of modern baby food. Then we'll look at best practices for starting solids—how, when, and what to feed infants. Beth and I will give you portion sizes, feeding guidelines, and sample meal plans to make it simple and easy to start solids the right way. My hope is that you'll see that the better choice for your baby is to make these foods at home, because the ultimate goal is to get your baby used to different flavors and textures in order to train his palate to desire real, whole, healthy foods.

The Case for Skipping the Baby-Food Aisle

Let's look at some of the factors that typically go into parents' decisions about whether to purchase store-bought baby food or make their own.

Ingredients and Nutritional Benefits of Baby Food

Countless feeding books and cookbooks will tell you that commercial baby food is filled with sugar, salt, and chemicals. You may be surprised to learn that this statement is not always true. *Some* commercial baby foods, such as those designated "first foods" (also commonly called "stage-one foods"), are actually good choices nutritionally, containing just one food, water, and perhaps vitamin C—no added sugar, salt, or chemicals.

To be honest with you, *nutritionally* there may not be much difference between a jar of stage-one bananas and home-pureed bananas. In other words, the vitamins, minerals, and calories will be very similar.

Yet some baby foods (especially those labeled "stage three," "toddler," or "graduate") do indeed have fillers such as sugar, salt, and various chemicals to stabilize and emulsify ingredients, and to extend shelf life. You might be surprised to learn that *some* commercial baby food available at your local grocery store (such as shelf-stable jarred food and baby teething biscuits) may be *older* than your actual baby!

For these reasons, I believe it's better to skip the baby-food aisle altogether and instead make healthy versions at home. However, I know this isn't always possible. If you choose to buy commercial baby food, my rule of thumb is that products for younger babies (stage-one foods) generally have fewer ingredients and are better choices. At the very minimum, make sure that each ingredient in a commercial baby food can actually be found in another area of your grocery store—no artificial or chemical additives.

Verdict: Not all commercial baby foods are filled with unhealthy ingredients, but some are, and should be avoided. Once a product starts going down the multi-ingredient road, its nutritional benefits drop compared to a homemade version. I suggest avoiding such products, with their yucky additives, and instead making these foods at home.

Texture and Variety of Baby Food

Have you noticed how each time you make a dish at home it turns out slightly different? At least it does in my house. Sometimes the meal turns out perfectly delicious, and sometimes . . . well, not so much. Produce that you buy at the grocery store also varies in taste depending on the season and ripeness.

In contrast, commercial processing results in uniformity in food. Jarred baby-food products always provide the same reliable but boring outcome: a uniform and very smooth texture and flavor. It's much better for an infant to experience the varying consistencies and tastes of home cooking and seasonal ingredients.

I find that parents who purchase large numbers of baby-food jars and pouches tend to keep their infants on these purees longer than necessary. Purees are needed for only a very short time, usually about eight weeks, depending on what age you start solids. Babies can rapidly advance to fork-mashed foods that are thicker, lumpier, and bumpier and usually healthier and easier if homemade.

Verdict: Commercial baby foods train children to expect sameness of flavor and texture, whereas homemade foods provide a variety of flavors and textures to tempt their blossoming palate.

The "Just for Kids" Mind-set and Baby Food

The most important reason to skip the baby-food aisle has nothing to do with nutrition. Go down the aisles of any major supermarket and you will see *thousands* of food products specially created for children, including animated character gummies, special yogurt with sprinkle toppings, sweetened waffle products, sugary cereals, dinosaur-shaped chicken, and more!

The mind-set that children eat separately from adults begins in babyhood. And it's dangerous! The most common complaint about childhood eating ("My child is *picky*!") is driven, at least in part, by these foods that are marketed to children. As kids accustomed to these foods grow older, they often don't recognize or aren't willing to try real foods. But you can prevent many future feeding problems by taking a different feeding path, as discussed throughout this book. And it starts by avoiding most of these "just for kids" foods.

Verdict: Foods that are created and marketed as "just for kids" may actually harm kids' healthy eating habits in the long run. Limit these products so that your kids learn to eat regular foods early on.

The Convenience of Baby Food

Let me see if I can read your mind. Right about now, you're probably saying, "But Dr. Tanya, commercial baby food is extremely convenient!" And you're right. It's especially helpful when your family is traveling or when you're busy. With commercial baby food you don't have to cook, wash pots, or defrost anything.

So let me put your mind at ease. I'm not saying that you should *never* purchase commercial baby food, just that you should limit it to when needed, such as when you're on a trip or have a week when you know you'll routinely be getting home late from work. If your Plan A is to make your own food the majority of the time, Plan B gives you the flexibility to buy healthy, commercial options when needed. When you *do* purchase commercial baby food, be sure to read ingredients and make nutritionally sound choices not only for your baby today, but also for her future life as a healthy, nutrition-loving, non-picky eater.

Verdict: We all have times when we need to go to Plan B and buy commercial baby food for the convenience it offers. Limit store-bought baby food to when needed, and always buy healthy options at the store.

The Financial Cost of Baby Food

Making your own baby food is *less* expensive than buying commercial products. At the store, you pay for the convenience; and if you want to buy premade *organic* baby food, you pay even more. Here are five tips for making homemade baby food at a very reasonable cost:

1. Cook food in bulk and freeze it in portions.

2. If buying food fresh, buy it in season.

3. Buy food on sale.

4. Buy frozen food, especially fruits and veggies.

5. Cook for your family and modify dishes for the baby. Many foods, including soups, casseroles, pasta dishes, and meats, can be easily modified/pureed.

Verdict: It's actually cheaper to make your own baby food than to buy jars or pouches at the store. In fact, three of the above tips are virtually identical to our time-saving tips in the section below. So you can have your baby food and eat it too, cutting down on both cost and time!

Baby Food for the Busy Parent: The Time Cost

The concept of "cost" does depend on the person. Time is money, and some people with very limited time will gladly pay a little bit more to enjoy the convenience that commercial products provide. Here are our top four ways to reduce the time involved in making your own baby food:

1. MY FAVORITE SOLUTION IS TO ENLIST A GRANDPARENT'S OR CAREGIVER'S HELP. Beth's neighbor Robin has a granddaughter who is now three years old. Her son and daughter-in-law are both busy working parents. Robin is a great cook, and when her granddaughter was younger, Robin helped out by making food for the baby. If you don't have a grandparent who can help with this, perhaps there's another relative or close friend who likes to cook and would be willing to pitch in.

2. COOK IN BATCHES. If a friend comes to visit, let him or her entertain the baby while you crank out a few batches of pureed carrots you can later freeze. Make a few servings of whole-grain pasta that can stay in the refrigerator for a few days. When you make scrambled eggs, make an extra portion for the next day's breakfast.

3. BUY FROZEN PRODUCE. Frozen produce without added sauces or preservatives is nutritious, convenient, and inexpensive. Keep

bags of frozen peas, green beans, broccoli, mixed veggies, berries, peaches, and more on hand.

4. ADAPT THE FAMILY MEAL FOR YOUR BABY. When you cook, keep a portion unseasoned (or plainer) for the youngest member of the family. Leave your baby-food blender or mini–food processor out on the counter so that you can easily blend what the rest of the family is eating at the table. As soon as your baby tolerates it, advance to fork-mashed food, then crumbled-up tiny pieces. By modifying family food, you aren't spending time making food for just one person.

Verdict: When time is precious and you find it challenging to make your own baby food, use time-saving tips like the ones listed above.

How to Make Your Own Baby Food

Weighing all these considerations side by side, it's easy to see that there are greater benefits to be gained by skipping the baby-food aisle and making your own foods at home, than by using commercial baby food. However, I also realize that every home is different, and you should determine the best way for *your* family to address this issue. Maybe you'll make all the baby food at home, or maybe you'll make just a few key foods. But the most important thing to remember is that home-prepared foods will help you build a bridge between "baby feeding" and "family feeding."

Your baby will see the whole process—see the bright yellow banana before it's mashed up, and maybe even share some of it with you. She will smell and taste natural variations, such as ripeness. Some of your home-made banana will be thinner and some will be lumpier, depending on how long you pureed or mashed it. All of these factors are important in teaching your infant to desire a variety of healthy tastes, consistencies, and smells. Making baby food at home will also make it easier for you to help your child advance from purees to mashed food, to small pieces, and later to self-feeding. What's more, I think you'll find making baby food much easier than you expected. Let's start simple in this chapter, but you can also turn to chapter 15, "Recipes," for more ideas!

Almost all baby-food recipes can be broken down into four simple steps as follows:

1. COOK/STEAM/BAKE. This step is for foods a baby can't eat raw, such as sweet potatoes, green beans, peas, white potatoes, broccoli, cauliflower, oatmeal, and carrots. Cook these foods the way you would cook something for yourself. This is very basic cooking—sticking a sweet potato into a 400-degree oven for an hour and baking it, for example, or steaming carrots or broccoli.

   There are shortcuts you can use. For example, my cousin works full-time and is making food for her second child. She uses organic canned green beans that she can puree at home, thus skipping the step of cooking green beans. Frozen produce is a lifesaver, too!

2. BLEND. My favorite tools for blending are a high-powered traditional blender and an immersion blender because you can continue to use them for years (even decades). Special baby-food appliances are often easy to use and clean, but may have less utility as kids grow.

   An immersion blender is handy because it goes right into the pot, meaning you skip the step of transferring food into a blender. An immersion blender is especially useful when making soups.

   A mini–food processor is also a useful tool. It takes up little room and is a cinch to use. You can throw regular oatmeal into it, turn it on, and in seconds have your own baby-food oatmeal that's super-smooth. You can throw in chunks of cooked potato, sweet potato, or carrots and have a smooth texture in seconds.

And last but not least, when your child can start eating lumpier and bumpier foods, I love my good old-fashioned potato masher!

BETH'S GROCERY GUIDE

Frozen vs. Canned vs. Fresh

Frozen: Did you know that sometimes frozen produce is actually superior to fresh? Some fresh produce is sold out of season (like nectarines grown far from home in February), or has deteriorated on a long journey from farm to store. Frozen produce, on the other hand, is often processed right after picking and thus retains very high nutritional quality. So stock up on frozen produce. It's easy to steam and puree; but best of all, it won't go bad in just a few days like fresh produce.

Canned: Canned food has come a long way in the past two hundred years. Certainly canning remains a healthy and convenient way to preserve food for long periods of time. Many parents express concerns about bisphenol A (BPA), a chemical used in the lining of some metal cans that may leach into canned food. Most studies I've seen have found widely varying levels of this chemical in canned foods, some low, some higher. Some companies are now selling canned beans and other foods in BPA-free containers, a positive trend. I don't recommend having canned food every day, but some canned foods (especially BPA-free, low-salt, organic options), used occasionally, provide a nutritious and convenient option.

Fresh: Fresh foods are actually a modern convenience! Hundreds and thousands of years ago people were slaves to weather and soil conditions, and a modern grocery store would have been unthinkable. We are so lucky to have a huge array of fresh products to choose from!

3. ADD LIQUID. Whatever appliance you are using to puree, you will probably need to add extra liquid to achieve the right consistency, especially when your baby is first starting solids and needs food very thin and smooth. While some foods such as zucchini can easily be pureed and served just as they are, many other foods, such as carrots, sweet potatoes, and chicken, need a little help from added liquid. Great options include water, breast milk, and healthy homemade or organic low-salt chicken or vegetable broth.

4. STORE AS DESIRED. Don't hesitate to make a big batch and store some for later. Leftovers can be used on their own or as add-ins. For example, extra pureed carrots and sweet potatoes, can be kept on hand to add texture and flavor to other foods.

   You don't need anything fancy here! The best option for storage is simple ice-cube trays. Transfer your purees to ice-cube trays, then freeze. After the blocks are frozen, pop them out and store them in freezer-safe bags or containers. As you need them, take out and thaw the frozen blocks.

Ten "Recipes" for Beyond-Easy Baby Food

Here are ten simple ideas to get you started. These ideas are all appropriate for babies starting around six months of age. (See chapter 15 for more baby- and family-friendly recipes.) Notice how my Eleven Foundation Foods are well represented in this list.

1. Fork-mash a banana. Thin the result with breast milk or water if desired.

2. Scramble an egg and puree or mash it up once cooked with extra liquid if needed.

3. Make vegetable, chicken, or lentil soup and pour some into a high-powered blender. Once it's pureed, pour the liquid into ice-cube trays and freeze. (See page 295 for a tasty lentil soup recipe.)
4. Bake a sweet potato for an hour, or until very soft. Fork-mash and thin the pulp with breast milk, chicken broth, or water, stirring until you reach the desired smooth consistency.
5. Put dry oatmeal into a mini–food processor and pulse it into tiny flakes. Cook the oatmeal as directed on the package, adding extra water if you want the result thinner.
6. Roast vegetables with olive oil and then puree them in a mini–food processor or blender with some chicken or vegetable broth.
7. Mash an avocado, thinning the mash with breast milk or water if desired.
8. Steam carrots until they're very soft, and then puree them to the desired consistency with extra water.
9. Buy cubed butternut squash and steam or bake it. Puree it in a blender or mini–food processor with extra water. Add a dash of cinnamon if desired.
10. Buy frozen or fresh berries and puree them in a blender or mini–food processor with a little bit of water.

The Infant Program

Now that you've had a great introduction to various baby-food options, with advice as to the best choices, let's talk about actually feeding your baby! Your baby has been on a liquid diet for months, and he's now starting to realize that there's more to life than just the breast. It's pretty exciting when he notices what *you're* eating and starts watching you like a hawk. Your baby's own interest in solid foods is a sign that he might be ready to start joining the family table.

Research shows that starting solids *before* four months of age can be linked to childhood obesity, while waiting until *after* six months can contribute to anemia. All babies grow and develop at different rates, so how do you know when your baby is ready to eat?

Around six months of age most babies become developmentally ready to start solids. Their head control improves and they become able to move solid food from the front to the back of their mouth with their tongue. Before this time, if you offer your baby a small spoonful of baby food he will simply push it back out at you. It's a reflex (the extrusion reflex) that disappears around six months of age.

You may also notice "readiness signals." For example, your baby may begin pulling off of your breast more, looking around; he may show interest in what you're eating; and he may put his hands in his mouth more often, bringing toys to his mouth and exploring everything by mouthing—yum! Around six months of age he will also be able to signal you when he wants a specific food by leaning forward and opening his mouth. When he's full (or doesn't like what he's been given), he will lean back or turn away.

The American Academy of Pediatrics and most pediatricians and feeding experts recommend starting solids around six months of age. The key word is "around." Every baby grows and develops at a different rate. Parents who think their baby is ready often ask me, "Can I start solids before six months?" The answer is often yes. Some babies can't wait to begin tasting solid food and can start as early as four months. If "readiness signals" are present in your baby at that young age, go ahead and try. If he pushes the food back at you with his tongue, wait another week or two and try again. However, if your baby is feeding well during the day, growing well, and sleeping through the night, you can wait until closer to six months to begin solids.

As a mom, I know it's exciting to begin feeding your baby, but go slowly and choose wisely. Your baby has his entire life to enjoy a wide range of foods. Below, I will give you tips on how to begin solids, a sample infant feeding schedule, portion size information, and advice on what age and stage a baby is ready for certain foods. Use this information to guide you as you determine how and when to start solid foods.

Tips on Beginning Solids

Choose a food and a time to start. (See the Sample Infant Feeding Schedule, found on pages 90–91, for guidance.) You will generally offer solid food just once a day at first. Here are my tips on starting solids:

- RELAX. Choose a relaxed time of day, when you're not rushed.
- FOCUS. The actual "feeding" will last less than fifteen minutes. Put your phone and all electronics on silent mode and tuck them away. Don't text and feed!
- HAVE FUN. Make mealtime fun for both of you, even when it gets messy—and it will.
- CHOOSE YOUR TIME WISELY. It's best if your baby is well rested. An hour or so after her nap often works best.
- START WITH ONCE DAILY. Once a day works best at first. Some babies will advance fairly quickly to two to three times a day, while others are happy eating once a day for a few weeks or more.
- WATCH FOR CUES. Let your baby signal you when to start and stop. She should meet you halfway, leaning forward eagerly in anticipation of the food. If she's leaning back with her mouth closed, don't force the spoon in. If she starts turning her head away, that's probably her way of telling you she's *done*! Don't try to get "just one more bite" in. Respect her fullness signals.
- REMEMBER THAT PRACTICE MAKES PERFECT. Most of your baby's calories are still coming from breast milk. Don't worry right now about the quantity of food she's eating. She is simply practicing (learning to eat) and tasting (exploring and getting used to a variety of healthy foundation foods).

M's Food Diary

Adventures in Starting Solids with My Third Boy

Every baby is different. My three boys all ended up starting solids at completely different times. I gave birth to my third in the middle of writing this book, so I kept a record of how I started solid food with him.

Four Months

M is nursing well and is alert and interested in what's going on in the house during the day. He can hold his head up well and push up on his tummy. He hasn't started rolling over and isn't yet paying attention to others in the family when we're eating. When I give him his vitamin D drops he pushes out his tongue and gags on the liquid. I was planning on starting solids around four months because he's bigger than my other boys were at that age, has good head control, and is very active, but now I see that he's not ready. I'll give him another few weeks and reevaluate.

Five Months

M is rolling! Back to front and front to back. Seems a bit more interested in *my* meals, so I decided to try some pureed avocado with breast milk. He held it in his mouth; he didn't push it out, but neither did he seem to know how to move it around in his mouth and swallow it. I'll wait another week.

Five and a Half Months

Beth made pureed organic vegetables, froze them in ice-cube-size trays, and brought them over for M. Now he has options: carrots, sweet potatoes, green beans, and broccoli, all pureed separately. He *loves* the carrots. After one bite he was excited about eating. Now he eagerly opens his mouth and easily moves the carrot puree from front to back and swallows it.

Over the course of a week we've advanced to two 1-ounce feedings a day of pureed veggies. As soon as I put him in the high chair, he wants to eat. I've never seen an infant so excited about veggies! Green or orange, he loves them all!

Six Months

I'm now wanting to get some iron and protein into M's diet. I bought whole-grain organic baby oatmeal, cooked up 1 ounce of it with breast milk—and he loved it! We've tried variations of oatmeal mixed with veggies, prunes, and even peanut butter. I melted 1 teaspoon of peanut butter into 1 ounce of oatmeal and added extra breast milk to make the mixture thin and not too sticky. He gobbled it down. While out with a friend's baby, we tried pureed hard-boiled egg (I added a little water to thin it) and plain whole-milk yogurt. He's on his way!

Seven Months

With encouragement from Grammie, we've slowly moved M up to eating three meals a day—typically oatmeal for breakfast, a veggie for lunch, and a chicken/veggie mix for dinner. Overall, I'm trying to get eggs, avocado, chicken, peanut butter oatmeal, plain yogurt, prunes, and a variety of green and orange veggies, fruits, and berries into him regularly. He's still eating purees, but sometimes I make them a bit thicker. He enjoys sips of water during meals from a bottle or straw. The last of the Eleven Foundation Foods to try . . . salmon!

Sample Infant Feeding Schedule

Food Category	Around 6 months	6 to 8 months
	Feeding Readiness: Sits supported, has good head control, is able to move food from front to back of mouth, does not push food out with tongue, is interested in eating, watches you eat, opens mouth to eat	**Feeding Readiness:** Sits alone, has good head control, is able to tolerate thicker or lumpier consistencies, mashes food with gums, is beginning to take sips of fluids from cup
Breast milk	About 6 times per day (generally 4–6 ounces each feeding)	6 times per day (generally 4–6 ounces each feeding)
Vegetables	Pureed, 1–2 tablespoons a few times a week	Pureed or mashed, 2 tablespoons once or twice a day
Fruit	Pureed, 1–2 tablespoons a few times a week	Pureed or mashed, 1–2 tablespoons once a day
Cereal/Grains	Infant cereal, 1 to 2 tablespoons a few times a week	Infant cereal, 2 tablespoons 3–4 times a week
Meat (including chicken) / fish / egg	Pureed chicken or meat, 1 tablespoon a few times a week	Pureed chicken, meat, or mashed cooked egg, 1–2 tablespoons 2–3 times a week
Yogurt/Cheese	A taste of yogurt once or twice a week	2 tablespoons yogurt 2–3 times a week
Water	Sips of water	Sips of water

8 to 10 months	10 to 12 months
Feeding Readiness: Sits alone well, palms and picks up food pieces, bites off pieces of food, moves food from side to side in mouth, drinks from sippy or straw cup	**Feeding Readiness:** Picks up small pieces of food well and self-feeds, chews better, drinks from cup
4 to 6 times per day (generally 4–8 ounces each feeding)	About 4 times per day (generally 6–8 ounces each feeding)
Pieces of soft-cooked or mashed, 2 tablespoons, 2 servings a day	Pieces of soft-cooked or mashed, 3 tablespoons, 2–3 servings a day
Pieces of soft-cooked or mashed, 2 tablespoons, 2 servings a day	Soft pieces or mashed, 3 tablespoons, 2–3 servings a day
2 tablespoons cereal or pasta or ¼ slice bread, 2 servings a day	2–4 tablespoons cereal or pasta or ¼ slice bread, 3 servings a day
Tiny pieces or mashed bits of moist lean meat, chicken, fish, egg, or cooked beans, 2 tablespoons 3–5 times a week	Tiny pieces or fork-mashed bits of moist lean meat, chicken, fish, egg, or cooked beans, 2 tablespoons 3–7 times a week
2–4 tablespoons yogurt, or 1 slice cheese, cut in small pieces 2–3 times a week	4 tablespoons yogurt, or 1 slice cheese, cut in small pieces 3–5 times a week
A few ounces a day	A few ounces twice a day

Safety Tip

Choking Hazards: Almost any food that is too big or too hard is a potential choking hazard.

Here is a list of unsafe foods for infants and toddlers:

- Whole nuts
- Grapes (unless cut in quarters)
- Popcorn
- Hot dogs (unless cut lengthwise, then sliced and quartered)
- Raw carrots (unless cooked until soft, then cut up)
- Cherry tomatoes (unless cut in quarters)
- Hard candies, including jelly beans
- Chunks of peanut butter (okay if spread thinly)
- Sunflower or pumpkin seeds
- Large chunks of any food, such as meat, fish, potatoes, raw vegetables, and raw fruits

Portion Sizes for Infants

Parents are often surprised when I discuss how tiny a baby's portions should be. Infants may start with just a teaspoon or two of something, then work their way up to 1 to 2 tablespoons a few weeks later. Always start small; you can certainly offer more. Here are some examples of portion sizes for a typical six- to twelve-month-old. All foods below should be pureed, mashed, or cut into appropriate sizes to prevent choking hazards.

⅓ egg

¼ slice soft wheat bread/toast

1 tablespoon chicken / red meat / fish

1 to 2 tablespoons fruit or vegetables

1 to 2 whole-grain crackers

1 tablespoon beans

1 tablespoon whole-grain pasta or brown rice

2 to 4 tablespoons cooked or dry whole-grain cereal

Liquid Measure Equivalents

1 cup = 8 ounces = 16 tablespoons = 240 milliliters

½ cup = 4 ounces = 8 tablespoons = 120 milliliters

¼ cup = 2 ounces = 4 tablespoons = 60 milliliters

⅛ cup = 1 ounce = 2 tablespoons = 30 milliliters

1 tablespoon = 3 teaspoons = 15 milliliters

Dry Measure Equivalents

½ cup = 8 tablespoons = 24 teaspoons

¼ cup = 4 tablespoons = 12 teaspoons

⅛ cup = 2 tablespoons = 6 teaspoons

1 tablespoon = 3 teaspoons

Infant Feeding: Ages and Stages

Age: Around six months

FOOD STAGE: Starter foods

BIG GOALS: Learn how to manage pureed consistencies; for parents, start training your baby's early palate

Introduce single-ingredient foods first. Try pureed vegetables, fruits, avocado, chicken, meat, and/or cereals. Meats and/or cereals should be introduced around six months, because breast-fed infants need extra iron and zinc at that age for proper growth and development. As soon as possible, at least one feeding per day should also contain foods rich in vitamin C, such as pureed green vegetables or pureed fruit. Whichever single-ingredient food you decide to introduce first—chicken, meat, cereal, or veggie/fruit—start with just one feeding a day and gradually work up to more.

To prepare a one-ingredient starting food, cook your chosen food until it's a soft consistency (just a little softer than you would want for yourself), then add breast milk or water and blend to the desired consistency. The puree should be soup-like so that it runs right off the spoon. Over time you can gradually make the consistency thicker.

➢ Dr. Tanya's Tip: Throw Out the Rice Cereal

Years ago, infant rice cereal was recommended as *the* first food for babies. It still has much to recommend about it. It's generally fortified with iron and zinc, which infants need around six months of age. It's also convenient, and most babies readily accept it. By changing the amount of liquid you add, you can alter the texture from soup-like to semisolid, making it suitable for a wide range of ages.

Not all cereals are created equal, however. More recently, white rice has been targeted by some experts as contributing to the obesity epidemic, because it has little nutrition. White rice contains little protein and no fiber, and its iron and zinc aren't as well absorbed as we'd previously thought. In addition, there is growing concern over arsenic in the soil in which our rice is grown. (See the Safety Tip on arsenic and rice on page 96.)

So what is a better early option? Meats! Meats (including chicken and turkey) are a great source of iron and zinc, and the iron and zinc in meat are better absorbed than those from cereal.

If you do choose to give your baby infant cereal, choose brown over white options: they are more nutritious, and they get your infant used to the taste of whole grains. Try brown rice, oatmeal, barley, quinoa, or wheat infant cereals. Remember that whole grains do provide a great source of nutrition to your child, especially in the coming years, including calories (energy), fiber, vitamin E, and the B vitamins. In addition, whole-grain cereals can be mixed into fruits, vegetable, meats, and other pureed baby foods to thicken the consistency when needed.

Safety Tip

Arsenic and Rice: Arsenic, an element that occurs both naturally and via human pollution, is found in many foods, including grains, fruits, and vegetables. It is absorbed by plants from the soil and water, regardless of whether crops are grown under conventional or organic farming practices. While most crops don't absorb significant amounts of arsenic, rice is different: it takes up arsenic from both soil and water more readily than other grains. That said, whole grains are part of a well-balanced diet. The key word is "part."

Here is what three expert organizations have to say about arsenic and infant rice cereal:

> *The American Academy of Pediatrics advises that parents offer their children a wide variety of foods, including other grains such as oats, wheat and barley, which will decrease their child's exposure to arsenic from rice.*[6]
>
> —From the American Academy of Pediatrics

> *To reduce arsenic risks, we recommend that babies eat no more than 1 serving of infant rice cereal per day on average. And their diets should include cereals made of wheat, oatmeal, or corn grits, which contain significantly lower levels of arsenic, according to federal information.*[7]
>
> —From *Consumer Reports*

> *The FDA is unaware of any data that shows a difference in the amount of arsenic found in organic rice versus non-organic rice.*[8]
>
> —From the U.S. Food and Drug Administration

Bottom line: if you do feed rice cereal, limit the servings to one a day for infants, and let go of the mentality that rice cereal needs to be the base of your baby's food pyramid.

➢ Dr. Tanya's Tip: The Other End

Many babies get constipated around the time solids are introduced. As noted earlier, prunes are *the* best food to help your baby have regular, consistent stools. Incorporate prunes into your baby's daily feeding schedule as a preventive measure, or offer them on an as-needed basis. Keep pureed or baby-food prunes on hand, because when your little one needs prunes, *you* need them ASAP!

Age: Six to eight months

FOOD STAGE: Gradually moving from pureed to fork-mashed and thicker foods, starting finger foods

BIG GOALS: Continue learning how to chew, learn to manage thicker, lumpier foods, and start drinking water; for parents, increase feedings to two a day and continue training your baby's taste buds

When your baby is this age, most of her calories will still come from liquid. Solids may start to take a greater role, but don't worry about the amounts she's consuming. Feed your baby twice a day with a variety of pureed fruits and veggies, mashed avocado, mashed banana, and pureed meats, beans, and/or cereal. Don't force your baby to eat. Let her signal you when she's ready to eat (by opening her mouth and leaning forward) and when she's full (by leaning back and turning away).

Once single-ingredient foods have been tried, advance to mixed-ingredient foods and to thicker or lumpier consistencies.

Safety Tip

Honey: *Never* give a baby under one year of age honey because of the risk of infant botulism, a deadly disease. Babies, unlike older children and adults, do not have the ability to fight the botulism toxin that can be contained in honey.

Increase Feeds to Twice a Day

Once your baby has enjoyed eating once a day for a few weeks, try taking him up to twice a day. You can offer him the same thing twice, or you can mix it up a bit with cereal and fruit for breakfast and a veggie and meat for lunch or dinner. Sample daily schedules for six- and eight-month-olds are shown below. Of course, *your* infant's schedule may vary, based on his appetite and how long he sleeps at night and at naptime.

Sample Daily Schedules

Six-month-old having mostly breast milk plus two small solid feedings daily

7:00 A.M. wake up, breast milk

9:30 A.M. breast milk and nap

11:30 A.M. 2 tablespoons green vegetable or whole-grain cereal, breast milk

2:30 P.M. breast milk and nap

5:00 P.M. 1 to 2 tablespoons pureed chicken and/or 1 to 2 tablespoons vegetable or fruit, breast milk

7:30 P.M. breast milk and bedtime

Additional breast-feeding as needed

Eight-month-old still having breast milk plus two to three bigger solid feedings daily

6:30 A.M. wake up, breast milk

8:00 A.M. breakfast: 1 to 2 tablespoons mashed banana, 1 to 2 tablespoons egg or yogurt and/or 2 tablespoons whole-grain cereal

9:30 A.M. breast milk and nap

11:30 A.M. lunch: 2 tablespoons green vegetable and/or 2 tablespoons chicken, fish, or beans

2:30 P.M. breast milk and nap

5:00 P.M. dinner: 1 to 2 tablespoons vegetable or fruit and/or 2 tablespoons soft whole-grain pasta

7:30 P.M. breast milk and bedtime

Additional breast-feeding as needed

Age: Nine to ten months

FOOD STAGE: Finger foods, soft mashed foods

BIG GOALS: Practice the pincer grasp, practice getting pieces of food from the high-chair tray to the mouth; for parents, choose *healthy* finger foods (not puffed cereal or snack pouches) and move toward three meals a day, working toward a more regular feeding schedule

➢ Dr. Tanya's Tip: Messy Is Good

It's okay if your baby makes a mess with food. That's half the fun! After all, mealtime is an important learning opportunity. Your baby is learning to enjoy healthy food. If you're worried about spilled carrots or stains from red-veggie pasta sauce, stick a washable mat under the high chair or feeding area (an old beach towel works too!). Or try "naked pasta night" and feed your baby with only his diaper on (bath to follow). That was a fun night in my house when my boys were young. I've had patients who created major food battles because they just didn't allow their babies to get dirty. Your baby is exploring food, and the job is messy!

By nine months of age, infants can usually chew and swallow more solid foods, such as pieces of soft vegetable or cooked whole-grain pasta. Between nine and ten months of age, most infants are able to pick up small pieces of soft food with their thumb and forefinger (the so-called pincer grasp) and can begin feeding themselves, but a combination of self-feeding and parent-led feeding is often needed to ensure proper nutrition. (For more about baby-led feeding, see chapter 13).

While puffed baby snacks are a good training food (easy to pick up and dissolve in the mouth), they aren't meant to be a major food source for your child; for example, those that are fruit- or veggie-flavored aren't meant to stand in for the real thing.

Better to offer small pieces of cut-up steamed veggies, beans, berries, and/or whole-grain bread or cereal—all make excellent snacks at home or on the go. For this age, I love the idea of the cute disposable place mats sold at baby stores. Lay a place mat down to create a clean surface anywhere and put small pieces of food (even tiny pieces of your own food) on it for your baby to pick up, smash, and enjoy eating.

Move toward feeding three times a day, and start thinking about timing meals with the rest of the family.

➢ Dr. Tanya's Tip: Baby's First Tooth

Your baby doesn't need teeth to be able to eat at this age. Babies eat by mashing the food with their gums, so even a toddler who doesn't get his first tooth until age one (like my second son) can still eat pureed, then lumpy food, and later small, soft pieces of finger food. That said, most infants do get their first tooth at six to eight months. (Beth's oldest daughter didn't get her first tooth until fourteen months, so don't worry if your infant's first tooth comes later than the average!) Whenever your child gets her first tooth, start caring for it by gently wiping it off or brushing it at night. A tiny smear of fluoride toothpaste on the toothbrush at night also helps protect new teeth from cavities and keep them healthy.

Sample Feeding Schedule

Ten-month-old having three regular solid feedings daily

6:30 A.M.	wake up, breast milk
7:30 A.M.	breakfast: 2 tablespoons egg, 2 tablespoons fruit
9:30 A.M.	breast milk and nap
11:30 A.M.	lunch: 2 tablespoons tiny pieces of chicken, 2 tablespoons green veggies, ¼ slice whole-grain bread
2:30 P.M.	breast milk and nap
5:30 P.M.	dinner: 2 tablespoons fish, 2 tablespoons tiny pieces of a vegetable, 1 to 2 tablespoons whole-grain pasta
7:30 P.M.	breast milk and bed

➢ Dr. Tanya's Tip: Herbs and Spice and All Things Nice

If your family prefers, or if it's in your culture to use spices such as basil, cinnamon, cumin, or turmeric, go ahead and try small amounts in food that your baby will share. Such spices and herbs are not only tasty additions, but many have health benefits.

Family Feeding

Start trying to time a meal or two so that your baby can eat when the rest of the family eats. For some families, dinner might be easiest; for others, maybe breakfast on weekends. Letting your baby sit in a high chair at the family meal allows her to watch the process of eating, and smell and see what you all are eating, and she may be tempted to try what you're having. See chapter 7 for more information on eating together as a family.

Age: Eleven to twelve months

FOOD STAGE: Pieces of soft foods, finger foods

BIG GOALS: Eat meals with the rest of the family, have three regular meals per day, enjoy healthy and nutrient-rich foods; for parents, avoid buying and offering juice and "kid" food

Now is the time to have your child start eating along with the rest of the family. You can begin to offer your child part of what's on your own plate. While lunch may be a more kid-friendly meal, dinner can be whatever you make for the rest of the family, as long as it's appropriate and not a choking hazard.

At this age, babies get a combination of healthy finger foods as well as soft or mashed foods, depending on their preference. While it's perfectly fine to offer pieces of food from your plate, remember that you're training your little one's palate, so try to avoid sugar, salt, and other additives that your infant doesn't need (and you really don't either). At the first taste of juice or fast food (with their added sugar and salt, respectively), your infant may get hooked, so delay juice and fast food as long as possible.

> ➢ Dr. Tanya's Tip: Two Spoons Are Better Than One
>
> **If your baby is grabbing at the spoon while you're trying to feed her, give her her own spoon. She may not make it to her mouth yet, but while she enjoys trying, you can ensure that the nutrients get in with *your* spoon.**

Sample Meal/Snack Ideas for Infants

This table can be adapted for a child of any age who is eating solid food regularly, as long as the texture and size of choices are appropriate. For example, a scrambled egg can be served mashed or as bite-size finger-food pieces, depending on your child's age. A banana can be anything from baby food to big food—your child will gradually advance from pureed, to fork-mashed, to small bite size. Breast milk can be incorporated with every meal or snack below, as appropriate. After age one, you can serve whole or reduced-fat milk with meals. Serve water throughout the day, based on age-appropriate recommendations given in the feeding chart on pages 90–91.

Important: Adjust all foods listed below to prevent choking—that is, cut foods into very small pieces. Grapes, for example, should be quartered.

Sample Breakfast Ideas

1. Whole-grain bread or toast pieces; scrambled egg
2. Oatmeal; cut or mashed berries
3. Whole-grain cereal; mashed banana
4. Yogurt; pureed or diced pears
5. French toast made with 100 percent whole-wheat bread, served bite-size; pureed or small pieces of grated apple

Sample Morning Snack Ideas

1. Yogurt
2. Mashed or small pieces of avocado
3. Peeled and quartered grapes
4. Pureed or cut-up cooked veggies; small cheese pieces
5. Cut or mashed berries

Sample Lunch Ideas

1. Chicken, pureed or diced; soft whole-grain pasta; pureed or small pieces of peeled plum or peach
2. Whole-grain bread, in pieces; nut butter (a thin smear); mashed or diced cooked carrots
3. Mashed beans; shredded cheese; diced tortilla; mashed avocado
4. Turkey pieces; bread pieces; orange/clementine sections cut up; mashed or soft whole peas
5. Yogurt; cut or mashed cooked edamame or tofu; cut or mashed berries

Sample Afternoon Snack Ideas

1. Whole-grain cracker pieces; string cheese pieces
2. Applesauce
3. Yogurt
4. Nut butter (a thin smear); diced or sliced banana
5. Whole-grain cereal; diced cucumbers

Sample Dinner Ideas

These are family dinner suggestions that you can adapt for the age of your child.

1. Salmon, mashed or in pieces; quinoa; roasted cauliflower, mashed or in pieces; applesauce or shaved apple
2. Roasted or grilled chicken, pureed or diced; sweet potatoes, mashed; broccoli, steamed and mashed or in tiny pieces
3. Turkey meatballs cut in small pieces; whole-grain pasta with marinara sauce; melon, mashed or diced

4. Cooked lentils, mashed or whole, or lentil soup; bread, in pieces; baked plum or apple, diced
5. Lean hamburger or turkey patty, diced or mashed; whole-grain bun in pieces; fresh tomato pieces; pineapple, mashed or diced

---

I loved watching how my boys would progress from eating purees, to fork-mashed foods, to tiny pieces of what I was eating. The expression on their faces of excitement from new flavors and textures was precious and with each bite I knew that I was exposing their palates to nutrient-rich foods and creating lifelong healthy, nutrition-loving eaters. Of course, each of my three boys progressed through the stages at different rates and had different appetites. My first was able to handle small pieces at eight months, where my third was still on purees at that age. Try not to compare your infant to siblings, cousins, or friends, and just focus on nutrient-rich choices and creating healthy habits.

Remember This

- Homemade baby food exposes infants to more flavor, texture, and variety than commercial products. Making your own food saves money, boosts nutrition, and expands your baby's palate for the future.
- Limit rice cereal. Rice cereal does not have to be the first food, as once thought, or even the base of your baby's food pyramid.
- Advance beyond purees as soon as your baby is ready.
- Let your baby see you eat. Expose even young babies to the food the rest of the family is eating.
- When your baby is full, stop feeding. Do not force your baby to eat a certain amount. Watch his signals carefully, as he will tell you when he's full.

5.

The Toddler Program

Adventures with Independent Eaters

Toddlerhood—is there a more fun or (at times) more frustrating age? This description is especially true when it comes to eating. I often ask parents to describe how their toddler eats in a few short words. Top responses include: picky, possessive, rejecting, adventurous, entertaining, slow as a snail, chaotic, and "two bites, then all done"!

My favorite summary about feeding toddlers comes from nutritionist Ellyn Satter: "All young children are more-or-less picky about food. What they eat one day, they don't the next. They eat a lot one day, little the next. . . . They warm up slowly to unfamiliar foods and may have to see, watch you eat, touch or taste a food (they put it in and take it out again) 15 or 20 (or even more) times before they learn to like it. Then they eat it sometimes and not others."[9]

That's a pretty brilliant way to sum up how young children eat. Yet let me reassure those of you currently in this stage (and those who will be there soon!): ride out this "just say no" stage while maintaining the proper division of responsibility in eating (more on this soon), and your kids will:

- Eat a wide variety of foods
- Eat with the rest of the family
- Drink water
- Form a healthy relationship toward food

Remember the story of Goldilocks? One bowl was too hot, one was too cool, and one was just right. As feeding goes, you want neither to be too hot (too dictatorial, harsh, and restrictive) nor too cool (too permissive, letting your toddler decide and guide feeding).

This chapter will help you feed "just right," allowing your toddler to test her independence and assert her preferences while you enforce reasonable structure and family feeding rules. In addition, in this chapter I will tackle the common toddler feeding problems I see in my office, as well as offer suggestions for smart snacks and for ways to involve your toddler in creating healthy meals.

The big goal for feeding toddlers should be the child's gradual progression to eating with the rest of the family. If your toddler spends the next two years eating her own separate foods at separate times at a separate table, you will find it really hard to reverse this habit later. Let's start by looking at exactly how to bring your toddler to the table.

The Toddler Table

Your toddler has made a big switch. Months ago he was drinking a mostly liquid diet, supplemented by small amounts of solids. Now that he is one to two years old, he should be eating three healthy solid-food meals and one to two snacks daily. Milk and/or water can be served along with food.

Many young toddlers love to eat table food, and so they should. They enjoy feeding themselves and eating what they see others around them eating. As a parent, you are your child's best role model, so show him that you love your fruit, veggies, protein, dairy products, whole grains, and water. Have fun with the whole eating process. The parent takes a bite, your toddler takes a bite, and so on. Even eating off your child's high-chair tray or plate (with his permission, of course) will help model that healthy food is yummy food.

By age one, your toddler should be completely off pureed foods and able to eat small pieces of food. As he nears eighteen months to two years, he should advance as much as possible when it comes to solids. Most foods are fine as long as they are cut into tiny pieces, somewhat moist, and not stringy or hard to chew.

Toddler Feeding Jobs

Did you know that both you and your toddler have a job to do? Satter calls this the "division of responsibility in feeding." It looks like this:

> *The parent's job is to prepare and offer food at appropriate times.*
> *The child's job is to decide whether to eat (or not), and decide how much to eat.*

You should stick with your job description and let your toddler stick with his. Here are two typical toddler-feeding scenarios I've seen in my practice.

Scenario 1

Toddler starts throwing a fit as soon as she is placed in the high chair. Parent puts grilled chicken, green beans, potatoes, and apple slices on the high-chair tray. Toddler screams and throws food on the floor. Parent pleads with toddler to please try just *one bite* of the yummy, yummy green beans. Parent begs for fifteen minutes. Toddler refuses time and again. Parent gives up and makes the toddler macaroni and cheese. Toddler takes two bites of macaroni and cheese.

Diagnosis: Neither person is doing the assigned job correctly.

Scenario 2

Toddler and family (whoever is present at the time) sit down to dinner together. Toddler is part of the mealtime, and he can be brought out of the high chair as soon as he is ready. All members of the family choose from a nice variety of options—grilled chicken, green beans, roasted potatoes, sliced fruit, and bread. Toddler takes one bite of a green bean, smashes his chicken into the tray, and sucks on a fruit slice. He is happy and content. The family has a nice dinner, talking about their day and enjoying their meal.

Diagnosis: Both people are doing their jobs and respecting each other.

Obviously, scenario 2 is more desirable, because the family provided appropriate foods but did not force the toddler to eat. The toddler was in charge of portions and determined which foods he wanted to eat from the selections provided.

Bottom line: do not force your child to eat; just provide healthy and balanced meals at appropriate times. Model eating healthy foods. You can certainly *encourage* your child to touch, like, or taste a food, but do not force. Put your energy into preparing and serving good meals on a reasonable schedule, and let your child be in charge of her own hunger and fullness signals. If you're worried that your child is truly refusing food and not getting enough nutrition, speak to your pediatrician. (See the discussions about picky eaters in chapter 14 and about underweight/overweight concerns in chapter 12.)

Toddler Snack Attacks

Toddlers have tiny tummies and therefore often need a snack to tide them over until the next meal. If not chosen wisely, however, snacks can add empty calories that your child doesn't need. They can fill up your toddler's tummy so he isn't hungry for nutritious meals.

I wish I had stock in fishy crackers. The genius company that makes them has tapped into the toddler brain completely. What's not to love? They're small, orange, cute, crunchy, and tasty. Thankfully, the leading brand has removed fake colors from its product, but fishy crackers are still not the best daily choice, because they're made from processed grains, which means they're low in fiber. (If you do buy them, get the whole-grain version that has 2 grams of fiber per serving.) I find myself telling parents daily: fishy crackers are *not* an everyday snack!

Remember that all food, including snacks, counts positively or negatively toward your child's overall diet. Examples of positive contributions are good protein, calcium, and other nutrients, and negative examples are sugar and other empty or unhealthy calories.

The best way to approach snacks is to make them nutrient-rich mini-meals. I like to take full advantage of any small chance to provide extra nutrition in a child's diet. Try small pieces of cut-up veggies, beans, berries, and raisins, or a bit of whole-grain cereal—all make excellent snacks at home or on the go.

Twenty Healthy Snack Ideas for Toddlers

Remember to serve all of the following snacks in portion sizes that a toddler can easily handle, chew, and swallow.

1. Clementine pieces
2. Sliced grapes

3. Sliced pears
4. Sliced apple with creamy nut butter
5. Small cubes of watermelon or other melon
6. Sunflower seeds (for older toddlers)
7. Single-serving yogurt (without any fake colors)
8. Yogurt tubes (can be frozen overnight and packed for an away-from-home snack)
9. Whole-grain crackers and string cheese
10. Leftover sandwich
11. Whole-grain crackers spread with cream cheese
12. Slices of turkey and cheese
13. Hummus and whole-wheat pita bread
14. Small pieces of soft vegetables (try Persian cucumbers or cooked baby carrots) with or without hummus
15. Banana
16. Avocado
17. Whole-wheat mini-bagel with cream cheese or nut butter
18. Natural applesauce (no sugar added)
19. Dry whole-grain cereal
20. Smoothie made with Greek yogurt and fresh or frozen fruit

> ➢ Dr. Tanya's Tip: **Milkaholics**
>
> **Some toddlers would rather *drink* their calories than eat them, as noted in chapter 3. Often when parents come to see me about a picky toddler with a bird-like appetite, it's because their toddler is drinking 30 or more ounces of milk daily, which fills her up and blunts her appetite for solids.**
>
> **Yes, milk is a very important source of nutrition (see chapter 3), but too many liquid calories can decrease a child's appetite for actual food. If this is the case with your toddler, decrease the amount of milk to no more than 16 to 20 ounces a day; and for kids over age two, decrease the percentage of fat in the milk to low-fat or nonfat milk.**

The Great Chase: Trying to Feed Unwilling Toddlers

Toddlers don't enjoy sitting still; they're very busy little people with important things to do! Sitting at the table for a leisurely dinner is pretty low on their list of exciting activities. Hence, desperate parents resort to techniques such as distracting their toddler by serving meals in front of the TV, chasing her around the house with food, or begging and pleading with her to eat.

Such distraction techniques are a *huge* red flag that the mealtime dynamic needs an overhaul. For a better toddler eating pattern, follow these four steps:

1. FOLLOW A SCHEDULE. Have a schedule for meals and snacks instead of allowing your toddler to graze all day or eat on demand. (See below for advice on Toddler Time Zones.)
2. SIT DOWN, BOTH OF YOU. Whenever possible, provide meals and snacks at the table while your child is sitting down.

3. KEEP MEALTIME SHORT. Do not drag out the meal/snack for very long. As soon as your toddler starts losing interest in eating, ask her if she is "all done"; and if so, end the current feeding.

4. STAY AWAY FROM SCREENS. If you have to use distraction techniques (turning on the television, propping up the iPad/iPhone, playing "here comes the airplane," or chasing the child around the house), chances are your toddler isn't really that hungry. If you're concerned that he truly isn't eating enough, discuss your worries with your pediatrician. Relax; don't distract! Your child will eventually eat. Rest assured, I've never seen an otherwise normal child starve himself.

If your child eats one green bean for lunch and is "all done," don't try to chase her around to fill up her tummy. Remember the division of responsibility? She's held up her end; now it's time for you to hold up yours. Your secret weapon is your consistent feeding schedule: soon enough there will be another scheduled snack or meal, with awesome foods served. Maybe she will eat *two* green beans next time! Remove the pressure from your meals, focus on the cooking/offering instead of the consuming, and mealtime will be more fun and relaxing.

Many parents worry that if they treat mealtime this casually, their child won't receive adequate food or nutrition. They'd rather their child ate crackers throughout the day than only a few bites of veggies or chicken at dinner. The good news is: there's an intuitive solution for this. I call it Toddler Time Zones, and that's what we'll dive into next.

Toddler Time Zones—Feeding Schedules

A consistent but flexible feeding schedule will help ensure that your child gets adequate nutrition. I like author Dina Rose's idea of "Eating Zones,"[10] which Beth adapted into our Toddler Time Zones, explained below. You can start experimenting with Toddler Time Zones when your child is around age two. Age one is probably too young, because

Safety Tip

Eating on the Go: With a busy family schedule, it's realistic to assume that some meals and snacks may have to be eaten on the go or away from home, but it's important to develop the habit of eating at the table as much as possible. Remember that food eaten in the car, without direct supervision, can be a huge choking risk. You can't reach your child immediately or even notice if she is choking. Choose on-the-go foods with caution, favoring options such as whole-grain dry cereal placed in a single-serve bag, a quarter of a healthy sandwich, or small pieces of diced fruit. Keep even snack food healthy and appropriate. And remember that young children get used to routines easily: don't start an unhealthy habit, such as snack crackers or treats every time your child gets in the car, or she will learn to expect and crave them.

children of that age find the concepts hard to understand, and they may not yet have a consistent nap schedule. Gradually start Toddler Time Zones as your child gets a little older.

The Problem. Many toddlers and parents get into a vicious circle that goes like this. The child eats hardly anything at a meal, then comes begging for crackers twenty minutes later. The parents give the toddler the snack because they worry that their child is hungry, but then the toddler fills up on "filler foods" (a granola bar, crackers, etc.) and doesn't eat well at the next meal. This can go on all day, every day.

The Fix. Set up Toddler Time Zones for meals and snacks. For example, Breakfast Zone might be from 7:00 to 8:00 A.M., Snack Zone from 9:00 to 10:00 A.M., Lunch Zone from 11:30 A.M. to 12:30 P.M., Snack Zone from 1:00 to 3:00 P.M., and Dinner Zone from 5:00 to 6:00 P.M. Food can be served anytime during a particular zone, because we parents need some flexibility in timing.

The rule then becomes: no grazing in between these Toddler Time Zones. If your toddler eats only a little for breakfast, that's fine, because Snack Zone is coming up soon. But if she comes asking for a snack thirty minutes after breakfast, tell her she needs to wait until Snack Zone to eat again. And you don't have to feel bad, because you can serve snack at the very beginning of Snack Zone (9:00 A.M., for example). If your toddler comes asking for a snack between zones, you can remind her about the next time she'll get to eat, which in every case should be coming up soon. You can have as many Toddler Time Zones for extra snacks as you need; however, most toddlers should be able to go at least an hour between Time Zones.

The Toddler Time Zone approach is meant to be freeing, not restrictive. It lessens the worry a parent has about a picky toddler, because another meal/snack will be served soon, at a scheduled time.

As much as possible, serve sit-down, scheduled snacks rather than grab-and-go snacks that the child carries around the house and eats while playing or watching television. When possible at meals, have an adult sit and eat something—preferably the same thing—with the child.

Dinner timing is more difficult. Young children often have early bedtimes and thus generally need to eat dinner earlier than adults prefer—often at 5:00 to 6:00 P.M. Sometimes a caregiver might feed the kids dinner before a parent gets home, which is fine. See chapter 7 for ideas on how to integrate family meals into a busy family schedule.

Getting Your Child to Try New Foods: Trial by the Dozens

Why do most kids like cupcakes the first time they try them, but not green beans? Why must they be exposed to broccoli twenty times but a cookie only once? Many kids will naturally gravitate toward sweet tastes, while some need adjusting to bitter tastes. Processed foods high in sugar, salt, and/or fat are (and were designed to be) like a fireworks

Kids in the Kitchen

One of the best things about toddlers is their enthusiasm for learning and trying new things, which means that you can find fun ways for them to interact with their food. If they enjoy mealtime, they're going to be happier eaters and will develop lifelong healthy eating habits. Here are some ideas to make food fun:

- COUNT. Toddlers love to count! Have your child guess how many slices you can make from the banana you're about to serve. Count the pieces of chicken or beans in a bowl. Dump a pile of blueberries onto a plate and have your child count them.
- USE COLOR. Name all the colors on a plate filled with tasty morsels. See if your toddler can think of two to three foods that are green.
- PERSONALIZE. If you use ketchup or any kind of dipping sauce, buy squeeze bottles with a small nozzle or pour your homemade dipping sauce into a squeeze bottle; then draw with it. I sometimes write my children's names on their plates or make shapes with ketchup, and my kids love it!
- CREATE. Experiment with presentation ideas for fruits and veggies. (You can find lots of ideas online.) You can make a palm tree with banana slices for the trunk and kiwi wedges for the leaves, for example. Or you can make a cute face with "O" cereal outlining the face shape, raisins for eyes, cut tomatoes for mouth, and shaved carrot shreds for hair. There's no limit to your creativity here. When your kids are old enough, have them see if they can make something too!
- RELAX. Be more relaxed with cooking. The first time you make a new dish, consider it a first draft. I always say, "Number one is a trial run." Laugh at kitchen disasters. If you're enjoying mealtime, your child will too.

BETH'S GROCERY GUIDE

Terrible Toddler Foods

When children become adept at eating solids, they don't need any special "baby" or "toddler" food products. As mentioned in the previous chapter, most "toddler" and "graduate" products have long ingredient lists with multiple sugar and sodium sources, as well as unpronounceable preservatives.

Instead of a specific "toddler" ravioli, make a dish of regular ravioli for lunch and serve it to the whole family, not just the child. Want "toddler" turkey and mashed potatoes? Make your own turkey and mashed potatoes for the family and keep the leftovers for snacks over the next couple days. You can also buy cute little divided plates to put the meal on.

There's one exception: special toddler foods come in handy when you're on the go or traveling, but make a point to serve real (and therefore healthier) foods at home.

show in your child's mouth—exciting and tempting. That's just the way it is. So keep the fireworks to a minimum and increase exposure to nutrient-rich foods.

But how should you encourage your child to try new foods? Should you have your child try what some people call a "no-thank-you bite," use subtler forms of persuasion, or just let your child decide on her own?

I suggest presenting your toddler and family with a nice variety of foods and letting the toddler choose among those foods. Serve new foods along with old favorites so that your child becomes less intimidated by or distrustful of new menus. For example, serve a new grilled fish with favorite mashed potatoes and a favorite fruit. Your toddler, watching you try the foods, will try them on his own time schedule. Encouragement ("Wow, this cucumber is so crunchy") is fine, but I do *not* recommend forcing a child to swallow food. Forcing even a bite violates your food job (remember that division of responsibility?) and creates a battle. It doesn't lead to great long-term outcomes, either, because the child becomes distrustful of the situation and anticipates a horrible taste.

If you haven't already started the routine of family meals, I encourage you to get into that habit now. See chapter 7 for more information, including suggestions on dealing with hectic schedules and other challenges to feeding children. Remember: a big part of children learning to like new foods is seeing their parents eating and enjoying them as well, so family meals go a long way in teaching good eating habits.

It can take at least a dozen times for a child to accept a new food, so don't get discouraged if your child doesn't take to something the first few tries. (See chapter 14 for more help with picky eaters.) You have to take the time to keep introducing the new food every day, and let your child see you eating it too. If *you* don't eat the broccoli, *she* won't eat the broccoli. Involve your kids in grocery shopping, picking a new vegetable for the family to try, washing it, and preparing or cooking it, depending on their age.

As suggested earlier, you can name foods after your kids—or let them come up with names like "Zoe's Zucchini" or "Collin's Cauliflower." You can encourage them to introduce and explain their chosen food at the family dinner, along these lines: "This is green; I helped buy it today," or "I picked this and we steamed it and then added lemon and butter." Activities such as these will help your kids feel like they have a personal investment in what they're eating, and proud that they're contributing to family meals.

To sum up, keep trying and trying, be patient, and do not force. I promise you that the food conundrum will eventually work out in favor of the healthy, colorful, nutrient-rich Eleven Foundation Foods.

➢ Dr. Tanya's Tip: Constipated Toddlers

Constipation can cause endless problems in toddlers. If it hurts, they won't go. They hold it in, which makes it hurt even more. Constipation can also really interfere with potty training. Correcting and preventing constipation are very important no matter what age your kids (or you) are. There are six fruits and four juices that are natural laxatives:

- **FRUITS:** prunes, plums, cherries, apricots, pears, and grapes
- **JUICES:** prune juice, apple juice, apricot nectar, and pear nectar

Remember that most of a fruit's fiber is in the skin, so if you can puree pieces of *whole* fruit or get your child to eat the skin with the fruit, she will get more healthy fiber to prevent and treat constipation. Among the above-listed juices, I find that prune juice works the best. (I know that I've advised you several times against offering your child juice, but specific juices are an exception if your child is constipated.) If your child won't drink prune juice, even after you tell her how yummy it is, mix one part prune juice with two parts apple juice.

Drinking plenty of water every day will help as well. Toddlers should drink 16 to 24 ounces of water a day. Often just increasing your child's water consumption will do wonders for her stool.

Be sure to include plenty of fiber in your family's daily diet. Vegetables such as cauliflower and broccoli have natural fiber that helps keep children regular. When making pancakes, waffles, or oatmeal, you can add extra oat bran to the mix. (Some commercial frozen waffles are available with oat bran too.) Choose breakfast cereals and breads with at least 3 grams of fiber per serving. Whole-wheat bread and tortillas are good choices as well. Look for high-fiber wafers or crackers—a few of these a day keep many constipated kids regular. You'll find that replacing snack food with healthier, higher-fiber options not only is more nutritious, but also will help with constipation.

Sample Meal and Snack Ideas for Toddlers

Sample Breakfast Ideas

1. Scrambled egg; whole-grain toast, in strips
2. Oatmeal; berries, in pieces
3. Whole-grain cereal; sliced banana
4. Peanut butter on whole-grain toast; cubed melon
5. French toast made with 100 percent whole-wheat bread, in pieces; diced apple

Sample Morning Snack Ideas

1. Greek yogurt
2. Diced apple; string cheese
3. Grapes, quartered or halved
4. Whole-grain crackers; cheese, in pieces
5. Berries, cut

Sample Lunch Ideas

1. Chicken, in pieces; brown rice; cooked diced zucchini
2. Whole-grain bread with nut butter; cooked diced carrots
3. Beans, shredded cheese, tortilla, and avocado, either rolled up as a mini-burrito or served separately
4. Turkey, cheese, and whole-grain bread, either separate on a plate or presented as a sandwich; orange/clementine sections
5. Lean ham or turkey slices (nitrate-free); edamame; berries

Sample Afternoon Snack Ideas

1. Whole-grain crackers and hummus; string cheese
2. Diced apples; cooked diced carrots

3. Yogurt; raisins
4. Nut butter; sliced banana
5. Whole-grain cereal; diced cucumbers

Sample Dinner Ideas

These are family dinner suggestions that you can adapt for the age of your child.

1. Pot roast made in a slow cooker, in pieces; potatoes and carrots (cooked with the roast), in pieces; orange slices
2. Roasted or grilled chicken, in pieces; brown rice; mashed sweet potatoes; broccoli, steamed soft and in pieces
3. Turkey meatballs, diced; whole-grain pasta; marinara sauce; cubed melon; soft-cooked carrots
4. Black beans, avocado, cheese, and tortilla, either wrapped as a mini-burrito or served separately; cut-up apricots
5. Lean hamburger, cut; whole-grain bun, cut; small pieces of cut-up veggies from the family salad; cooked corn

---

If you follow our advice about the Toddler Time Zones, and regularly incorporate the Eleven Foundation Foods, your toddler's nutrition should be terrific. You will face other battles during these years that don't involve eating and nutrition. You'll find that the principles we advocate here apply in other matters as well. *Model good behavior* (eating healthy food), *involve your toddler* in choosing (healthy snack A or B) and creating foods, *make things fun* (eating with the rest of the family), and *keep consistently trying* (a dozen times or more).

Your job is to prepare and offer nutritious food at appropriate times. Your toddler's job is to decide whether or not, and how much, to eat.

Using Toddler Time Zones will help you ensure that your child eats enough nutrition at appropriate times throughout the day.

Remember This

- The big goal for feeding toddlers should be the child's gradual progression to eating with the rest of the family.
- Maintain the appropriate division of responsibility. The parent's job is to prepare and offer the food; the toddler's job is to decide whether and how much to eat.
- Set up a flexible feeding schedule using Toddler Time Zones. That way, if your toddler doesn't eat at one meal, you'll *both* know that another snack or meal is coming up soon.
- Don't chase, beg, bribe, or bargain with your toddler. This does more harm than good. Your toddler will eat when he is ready.
- Choose healthy snacks, not just fishy crackers!
- Milk has important nutrients. Toddlers should be drinking up to 20 ounces a day.
- Don't lose hope when introducing new foods. It can take at least a dozen tries for a toddler to accept a new food—unless it's a cookie.

6.

The Preschooler Program

Helping at Home and Lunchbox Lessons

Compared to mealtime adventures in the toddler years, feeding a preschooler is smooth sailing! Feeding becomes easier and more enjoyable as the older child becomes better able to help feed himself, use utensils, vocalize his preferences, and enjoy different textures and types of food. Mealtime can become a little calmer, as well, because the older child has a longer attention span and is usually somewhat more flexible. The big goals for preschoolers are that they should be eating healthy food at school and choosing real food at home (and school), instead of too much "kid" food.

Continue the idea behind Toddler Time Zones for your older child—that is, try to provide *scheduled* snacks and meals rather than giving them on demand. You can begin to guide your preschooler into a more structured feeding schedule that consists of three meals and two or three snacks daily. From preschool through elementary school, the model is generally as follows:

- Breakfast
- Morning snack, in conjunction with recess or playtime
- Lunch
- Afternoon snack
- Dinner
- Optional before-bed snack

Many kids this age will start giving up their nap and start attending preschool or kindergarten daily. This can actually make it easier to keep a consistent feeding schedule. I highly recommend an early dinnertime and early bedtime for this age group, especially when they stop napping. Many preschoolers do well eating dinner at 5:00 or 6:00 P.M., if you can make that work for your family.

For the breakdown of what to feed your child and when, refer back to the Preschooler Program section of chapter 2. Below we'll explore two important areas to focus on when teaching your preschooler healthy eating habits: eating at home, and eating at school. We'll include fun ways to include your child in meal planning and prep and eating, help you avoid picky-eating pitfalls, and give advice about how to pack nutritious school lunches that your kids will be excited to eat!

Kids at Home: Involving Your Child at Mealtime

As your kids get older, it becomes easier and more fun to involve them in the cooking and meal-prep process. Your preschooler has a longer attention span, can complete simple but fun tasks with you in the kitchen, and may be interested in learning about unfamiliar foods. There's a nutritional benefit to that involvement: kids are more likely to eat foods that they've helped prepare.

Use these creative ideas, and your own inspiration, to bring your preschooler into the kitchen:

Let Your Child Help You Cook

There are hundreds of ways an older child can start helping in the kitchen; here are ten fun ideas to get you started. Your child can:

1. Put toppings on her own pizza.
2. Skewer her own fruit. (We used to keep the long sticks used in delivered fruit arrangements to make it fun to eat fruit.)
3. Make her own healthy popsicles (see recipe on page 304).
4. Whisk eggs.
5. Shred lettuce with her hands.
6. Smash things! Graham crackers (for crusts or as parfait ingredients) and nuts or whole-grain cereal can go into a resealable bag, perfect for little hands to mash and crush.
7. Help measure dry ingredients.
8. Pour liquid ingredients into a bowl.
9. Make a menu, drawing pictures of the foods that will be served at the meal. This is a great distraction for while you are cooking!
10. Decide which dishes and utensils are needed for eating—plate or bowl? fork or spoon?—and help set the table.

Tip: Make it easy for kids by keeping a stepstool in the kitchen, or let them "cook" at a low kids' table.

Teach Your Child Simple Chores

There are different philosophies about when to start having children help out with chores around the house, but allowing your children to assist with simple tasks is often fun for them and helps them feel like they're contributing to the family. Here are a few ways you can involve your preschooler:

- Reorganize an easy-to-reach drawer or cabinet to hold kid-friendly bowls, cups, and plates so that your child can start choosing her own at mealtimes.
- Buy or make cute washable place mats your child can put on the table. We had place mats that taught the alphabet, counting, colors, and (later on) basic math facts.
- Start teaching your child how to clear her plate from the table when she's finished with her meal.

Teach Your Child Mealtime Manners

Even before the preschool years you should model appropriate manners to your child, but now that he's older it's time to start teaching and expecting certain basic mealtime behaviors. Remember that simple positive reinforcement is the best tool! Say, for example, "I love the way you put your napkin in your lap like a big boy!" Here are a few ideas to get you started on improving mealtime manners:

- Turn off or silence and put away all screens and phones at mealtimes. That goes for parents too!
- Teach your preschooler to use a napkin (not a hand or a shirt).
- Teach her to use a fork and spoon properly.
- Teach her an appropriate way to say that she doesn't care for a certain food, or simply to sit quietly after taking an unappealing

bite. I have a friend with a great catchphrase: "Don't yuck my yum!" When we're all at the table and she hears a kid (or adult) say, "I hate that," or "Eww, that broccoli is disgusting," she'll respond with, "Don't yuck my yum!"

Involve Your Child in Mealtime Conversations

Mealtime is a perfect opportunity for you to start learning what's going on in your child's life, and for her to start learning what the rest of the family is up to—so enjoy conversations with her. Teach kids that mealtime isn't just about eating. It's also a time to be together as a family and talk, not just shovel down their food and run off to play.

Teach Simple Nutrition Lessons

From grocery shopping to prepping and serving foods, you can create a nutrition lesson almost anywhere. This is a preschooler we're dealing with, so keep the explanations short and sweet: colors, food groups, and the importance of building healthy, strong bones.

- At this age, your child still respects your opinion. Start to teach her that "you are what you eat."
- At the grocery store, demonstrate how to count ingredients on a food label.
- Challenge your preschooler to pick out fruits and veggies of various colors. See if she can find something red, something green, and something blue, for example.
- At home, talk about the nutrition in the foods you're eating and get her used to recognizing the Eleven Foundation Foods.

> ➢ Dr. Tanya's Tip: **Start a Snack Box**
>
> **Make a box or bin of healthy items your child can choose from at snack-time. Pantry snacks might include whole-grain crackers, natural apple-sauce, natural fruit leather, raisins, nuts, and dried cereal. Refrigerated snacks could include yogurt tubes, fruit and berries, cut-up vegetables, small milk or chocolate milk cartons, and cheese sticks.**

Preventing Feeding Pitfalls

The most common complaint from parents about preschoolers is picky eating. And it isn't just the nuisance factor: if a child prefers to eat the same few foods daily, parents may worry that he isn't eating enough variety to get the range of nutrition he needs. We'll talk more about how to address picky eaters in chapter 14, but use the following six tips to prevent preschool-age feeding pitfalls.

1. Feeding is a marathon, not a sprint. Focus your energy on guiding long-term behaviors rather than short-term food choices. Do not count the green beans or fruit slices your child eats. Focus instead on providing healthy meals.
2. Avoid the job of short-order cook. You will have the best results if you make (or a caregiver makes) one meal for everyone, with individuals choosing which components they want to eat.

Family Feeding

Nuts and nut butters are easy to eat and require hardly any preparation. As a mom, I have snacks in my car, in my baby bag, and in every purse I own. A small bag of almonds is a great snack that keeps well, takes up hardly any space, and is ready when the kids say, "Mommy, I'm hungry!"

3. Keep your home a safe zone. You may have done an excellent job of shielding your child from juice, birthday cake, and piñata candy, but exposure increases at this age as he attends more birthday parties and playdates. It's important to keep the food in your house healthy and simple—save the juice boxes and candy for parties and playdates.
4. Keep offering different and new foods even if your child rejects them at first glance. Kids this age are still often very reluctant to try new things and—remember—it can take more than a dozen attempts for a child to accept a new food.
5. Ask yourself what *you* want to make and serve for dinner, *not* what your child wants to eat or will eat. Think of feeding as a tree. The parents or caregivers are on the top of the tree, *not* the child. What do *you* want to cook and serve for dinner? You don't need to ask what your child wants to eat: the answer will always be the same!
6. Keep buying one-ingredient foods (and packaged foods with short ingredient lists), and regularly offer all Eleven Foundation Foods.

Kids at School: School Lunch Lessons

At age four to five, many children start taking their lunch to preschool or even to early kindergarten. As they grow older, they will eventually consume 50 percent of their calories away from home (primarily during school hours). That's why it's vitally important to pack the right foods in your child's lunchbox.

You'll soon discover that lunchboxes run the spectrum between total junk and extreme health food. Should you send cookies or kale? Gummies or grapes? What you send depends on your beliefs, budget, and taste buds. Make lunch food desirable enough to entice your child

Cooking Help Desk

The Big Freeze: I love making healthy mini-muffins to send with lunch, but they quickly go stale. After the first day freeze the extras, first wrapping them well in plastic wrap or foil. Pack a frozen mini-muffin in your child's lunchbox. It will thaw by lunchtime, and your child will have a much better (and tastier) option than store-bought baked goods.

to eat it, without compromising on the necessities (all healthy food groups included, no fake colors, and 3 grams of fiber or more per grain item in the lunchbox). Sometimes parents pack too much food and almost all of it comes back uneaten. If your child has a small appetite, pack less—perhaps just three items instead of five.

Lunchbox Food Ideas: Cold Lunches

- Turkey slices, whole-grain crackers, carrot sticks, nectarine pieces
- Nut butter sandwich, cucumber slices, watermelon cubes, pretzels
- Turkey or other lean meat on whole-grain bread, apple slices, cut-up celery and carrots, healthy applesauce
- Yogurt (no fake colors), cut-up fruit, sliced carrots, whole-grain crackers
- Yogurt tube (frozen beforehand), sliced pear, sliced turkey, whole-grain pita bread
- Cold whole-grain pasta salad, watermelon cubes, cucumber slices, homemade oatmeal cookie
- Turkey sandwich or wrap, orange, fig bar, sliced bell peppers
- Whole-wheat mini-bagel with cream cheese, raisins, string cheese, sugar snap peas

- Chocolate milk, melon cubes, turkey slices, carrots with hummus or ranch dip, healthy baked chips

Lunchbox Food Ideas: Hot Lunches

To keep food hot, use a small Thermos-type bottle or other well-insulated container. In the morning, when you're preparing lunch, heat some water in a glass measuring cup for two minutes. Pour heated water into the insulated bottle, cover the bottle with its cap, and let it stand a few minutes. Then remove the cap, pour the water out, put the hot food in, and recap the bottle. That extra step will help keep your child's lunch hot until lunchtime.

Put in heated items such as the following:

- Quesadilla pieces
- Leftover pizza
- Turkey burger or garden burger
- Whole-grain pasta

Add fresh fruit, cut-up vegetables, a cheese stick, or yogurt to your child's lunchbox to round out the meal.

BETH'S GROCERY GUIDE

Pantry Produce

I keep "pantry produce" in the house as a backup for when I run out of fresh fruits and veggies. I like to stock natural applesauce, raisins, canned peaches, and dried fruit strips. Freeze-dried apples are also a great choice. If you send canned fruit with your child for lunch, give it a quick rinse (to wash off syrup or sugar) and then repack it in your own container.

Q&A: Solutions for Real Parent Questions

School Lunches

Q: My child wants a treat in her lunchbox every day. Is that okay?

A: It's fine, as long as it's a *small* treat—this could be a mini-cookie or mini-muffin (homemade), a single chocolate piece, or fruit gummies. Yes, packaged fruit gummies count as a treat, not a fruit!

Q: How bad are the fruit gummies my child loves?

A: As noted in the previous answer, fruit gummies with fun shapes really belong in the treat category, not the fruit category. Organic versions are certainly better because they don't have fake colors, but they're still a treat. Many brands have more than ten ingredients, and they're sweetened with fruit-juice concentrate. If you absolutely have to buy gummies, please don't buy a brand with fake colors!

Q: When should I involve my child in packing his lunchbox?

A: As young as toddler age, let him participate in choosing and helping to make his lunch. You can give him a choice of two acceptable items per category. For example, "Would you like turkey or nut butter on whole-wheat bread?" "Would you like string cheese or raisins?" "Would you like regular yogurt or a yogurt tube?" Let him put each item in his lunchbox.

Q: What are some good fruit options for lunches?

A: Include fresh fruit whenever possible in your child's lunchbox. Grapes, clementine pieces, and sliced apple are all good options that don't get squished. Cut-up melon and berries are great in sturdy reusable containers.

Q: My child refuses to eat any fruits or vegetables in her lunch. Help!

A: Even if your child doesn't eat fruits or veggies, include a bite or two in the lunch when you can, in the spirit of optimism. If it isn't in there, there's definitely no chance she'll eat it. Even if it's just a piece of watermelon, one cucumber slice, or one baby carrot, it's good to include *something*. The more your child is exposed to fruits and veggies, the more likely she is to eventually eat and like them.

Age Five and Beyond: Raising a Healthy Eater

Focusing on the grams, nutrients, antioxidants, and minerals going into your child is a recipe for frustration. Focus instead on forming good habits, serving great food, making mealtime a fun shared experience with your child, cooking *with* your child, setting a reasonable schedule for meals and snacks, and enjoying the Eleven Foundation Foods.

Kids are unpredictable, and their eating habits change with the wind. Your child's single-day nutrient consumption won't determine his future health. Feeding healthy kids is more like a marathon than a sprint, as noted earlier: you have a long way to go and plenty of time.

Safety Tip

When to Call the Pediatrician for Tummy Aches: The following signs indicate that your child's tummy ache needs to be evaluated by a medical professional right away; this means call your pediatrician *now* or go to the emergency room:

- Your child *looks* sick.
- The pain is worsening, severe, or constant for more than two hours (especially in the lower right side).
- Your child's belly is swollen, distended, or tender.
- Your child isn't interested in eating his favorite food.
- Your child is experiencing persistent vomiting or diarrhea.
- Your child has bloody, dark, or grape jelly–looking poop.
- Your child can't jump up and down without pain, can't walk, or walks hunched over.

➢ Dr. Tanya's Tip: Tummy Aches

As long as the pain isn't severe, worsening, or interfering with activity, you can take some time to assess the situation when your preschooler develops a tummy ache. If the discomfort lasts on and off for several days, watch for clues and patterns. Here are some things to think about:

- Is the pain related to any specific food or drink?
- Is it better or worse after eating or going to the bathroom?
- Is your child's stool regular, hard, soft, big, or small?
- How long and often has the pain been present?
- Where is the pain?
- Does the pain wake your child up at night or interfere with activities?
- Is the pain accompanied by vomiting, diarrhea, or fever?

It's often useful to keep a tummy-ache diary for a few days before you see your pediatrician. The diary should include what your child eats and drinks, when the pain occurs, what your child is doing at the time the pain occurs, how long the pain lasts, and (most important) how often your child poops and what it looks like.

There is no perfect way to help soothe a tummy ache. Some parents find that giving infants simethicone or other infant gas drops may help their gassy baby. For older infants and toddlers, a warm bath will bring some relief. Probiotics once or twice a day often help infants and children with tummy aches (adults too!). For more information on probiotics, see page 20. In addition, sips of peppermint or chamomile tea can soothe stomach aches.

Sample Meal and Snack Ideas for Preschoolers

Sample Breakfast Ideas

1. Whole-grain bagel with cream cheese or peanut butter; hard-boiled egg, cut
2. Greek yogurt, granola, and fruit parfait
3. Whole-grain cereal with milk
4. Scrambled or sunny-side-up eggs; whole-grain bread
5. Homemade blueberry muffin (see recipe on page 281); fruit

Sample Morning Snack Ideas

1. Yogurt and berries
2. Cottage cheese; fruit
3. Whole-grain crackers; cheese
4. Grapes; whole-grain dry cereal
5. Berry smoothie made with Greek yogurt (see recipe on page 303)

Sample Lunch Ideas

1. Turkey and cheese sandwich or rolled up in a tortilla; mango, cut; sugar snap peas, cooked
2. Whole-grain bread; nut butter; cucumber, cut
3. Tuna and whole-grain bread/crackers, served separately or as a sandwich; banana
4. Chicken, cut; brown rice; orange/clementine sections; asparagus, cooked
5. Bagel sandwich with turkey and cream cheese; melon, cubed; jicama, sliced into thin spears

Sample Afternoon Snack Ideas

1. Whole-grain crackers; string cheese
2. Celery with peanut butter
3. Yogurt; raisins
4. Apple slices with nut butter
5. Hummus with veggies or whole-grain pita

Sample Dinner Ideas

These are family dinner suggestions that you can adapt for the age of your child.

1. Turkey burger with sweet potato fries; watermelon, cubed
2. Quinoa pasta with marinara sauce; sunflower seeds; peas
3. Turkey meatloaf; squash, cooked and sliced or cubed; whole-grain bread; baked apple
4. Homemade pizza with healthy toppings like tomato-veggie sauce and cheese; mango, sliced
5. Chicken noodle soup; crusty whole-grain bread; carrots, cooked; blueberries

---

As noted earlier, during the preschool years your children will begin eating more and more of their calories outside of the "safe zone" of your home. Preschool, playdates, and birthday parties provide many opportunities for empty and unhealthy calories. Remember to use every opportunity you have to feed your child (and pack for your child) nutrient-rich meals and snacks. It may take a little planning, but it's completely doable.

Involve your child. Preschoolers love to "play chef" both in the playroom and with you in the kitchen. Use that to your advantage and begin to teach your child about nutrition, food groups, cooking, and the Eleven Foundation Foods.

I'll say it again—feeding healthy kids is more like a marathon than a sprint; you have a long way to go and plenty of time. But remember: what you instill in your preschooler she will remember and build on for years to come.

Remember This

- Keep in mind that the big goal for preschoolers is to eat healthy food at home and choose real food at school, rather than relying on "kid" food.
- Follow a structured meal and snack schedule to provide your child with needed calories; don't let your child graze the entire day.
- Let your child help you in the kitchen—your own little sous chef!
- Make your home a sugar-safe zone. Save the juice boxes and candy for birthday parties and playdates away from home.
- Don't be a short-order cook; make one meal for the whole family.
- Keep buying and offering one-ingredient foods, especially the Eleven Foundation Foods.
- Stock the lunchbox with healthy choices. Fifty percent of your child's calories will be consumed away from home once she starts school.

7.

The Modern Family Meal

Kids Eat Better When the Family Is Together

For much of human history, people had to cook in order to feed their family, and families had to come together to eat the food while the food was hot. Cooking was a requirement, not an option. Now many families rely on fast-food restaurants and supermarket deli counters. Our modern world is also different when it comes to schedules. Many families have an atypical schedule—perhaps you have a single-parent family, or shared custody, or you or your spouse or partner works late, or a caregiver serves dinner most nights. As a result of all these changes, meals eaten as a family aren't traditional anymore.

Even though our schedules are hectic and it isn't always possible to eat meals together, family dinners are extremely important. Studies show that families who eat dinner together actually have better communication, lower rates of obesity, and fewer picky eaters.[11]

Another recent study found that "family dinner was associated with healthful dietary intake patterns, including more fruits and vegetables, less fried food and soda, less saturated and trans fat, lower glycemic load, more fiber and [more] micronutrients from food."[12] Kids eat better when the family eats together!

The benefits don't stop at dinner. I encourage all parents to make mealtime with their family a priority. Remember: no Mommy (or Daddy) Guilt here! I believe that whatever your schedule or cooking experience, the modern family meal can be enjoyable, relaxing, flexible, and—most important—healthy.

For my family, with two working parents and busy boys in sports, music, and other activities, it's hard for us to eat dinner together every night. Nonetheless, we've worked together to carve out time for family meals. We use a mix of weeknights and weekends, dinner and breakfast, or even partial meals where we have family time to talk. Weekends often work better for us. We have more time then for family breakfast (my boys call it "special breakfast" because I really cook—healthy French toast or pancakes along with eggs and fruit). We also have "Daddy barbecue night," when my husband grills chicken or turkey burgers and the boys and I make veggies, brown rice, or other side dishes. Family lunch also often works nicely on the weekend, after a morning soccer game or before an afternoon activity. On weeknights that we don't have time for a full family meal together, the kids will often eat fruit and/or yogurt for dessert about an hour after their dinner or before bed, while my husband and I eat dinner. It's our own version of a modern family meal, allowing us still to sit and talk and eat together.

Beth's family meals look a little different, even though they're just as important. Her family also has two working parents, and they have two busy kids. Her husband often has an hour-long commute and gets home late many weeknights. The girls and Beth eat between 5:00 and 6:00 P.M. most school nights, all sitting at the table together. They have tasks and traditions: the girls help set the table and help clear their plates after eating, and they all go around the table talking about the best parts of their day and any problems they had. For them, this works better than feeding the kids early and the adults separately. On weekends they're more often *all four* at the table. They love weekend breakfasts together if they aren't running out to activities. Beth tries to make Sunday dinners a family tradition as well, and often invites friends and family. She has gotten fifteen-minute meals down to a science for weeknights. Her philosophy is "Keep it simple," and I agree! Below, we've come up with a few easy rules to keep mealtimes simple . . . and super!

The KISS Family Mealtime Rules (Keep It Super and Simple)

When it comes down to it, there are just a few attributes that are important for the family meal. They can be consolidated into three super and simple rules:

1. Everyone is eating the same foods. This exposes children to different foods, and parents aren't subject to short-order, picky-eating cooking.
2. Everyone is sitting at the table, which emphasizes the importance of togetherness in a harried and busy world.
3. Mealtime is free from electronics: no cell phones, emailing, or texting by anyone, parents included!

Rules that are deliberately missing from this list? Nowhere does it say you need to slave over a stove for hours. You don't have to be a gourmet chef or use expensive ingredients. Even if you get takeout and simply add a vegetable and fruit, you can still fulfill these three basic rules.

You can strive for the attributes of a family meal at any time—breakfast, lunch, or dinner. If you're not always home for a family dinner, don't despair. Instead, develop meal routines for other times of day.

For example, maybe you can eat breakfast together on weekdays, or have a big family lunch or dinner on weekends.

Many modern parents have limited cooking experience and are truly baffled and frustrated when they try to think of good meal ideas. Use the following five guidelines when you're planning a meal:

1. Serve a few different food groups: usually a protein, a starch/grain, one or more berries and/or vegetables, and some kind of liquid (water or milk). Make sure to include at least one or two of the Eleven Foundation Foods as well. Examples:

   Whole-grain cereal + milk + fruit

   Turkey/chicken sandwich + carrot sticks + pretzels + water

   Bean and cheese burrito + fruit + milk

2. Serve new experiments (like fish or lasagna) with old favorites (like bread or milk).

3. After age one, think of meal-making as a tree, as suggested in the previous chapter. The parent is at the top of the tree: What does the *parent* want to serve and eat? Then adapt the kids into the tree, perhaps cutting the food into small pieces for them, adding extra broth to their portions, and adding spices separately at the table so that children can decline if they want.

4. Ask your children for input, but limit them to two choices: Would you like to have sliced bananas or apples tonight? Should I make broccoli or green beans? Do you want sweet potatoes mashed or baked?

5. Have "Kids' Choice" night one to two times a week. At my house, "Kids' Choice" happens when the babysitter is there, I'm working late, or I'm having a crazy day and need a break.

Simple and Super Meals

Your family meals can be extremely simple, as shown in the ideas below. You can throw a preroasted grocery-store chicken on the table with bagged salad, fruit, and whole-grain bread in five minutes flat! And remember to include at least one or two of the Eleven Foundation Foods in every meal, which are well represented in the list below.

Ten Family Breakfast Menus

1. Cold whole-grain cereal + milk + sliced banana
2. Whole-grain waffles + nut butter + apple chunks
3. Oatmeal + chopped nuts + raisins/prunes + milk
4. Eggs + whole-wheat toast + pears
5. Vegetable scrambled eggs, egg frittata, or omelet + turkey bacon + whole-grain English muffins
6. Whole-wheat bagel + cream cheese or peanut butter + grapes
7. Greek yogurt + berries + whole-grain cereal
8. Scrambled eggs + tortilla + beans + avocado
9. Pancakes + raisins + milk
10. Whole-grain French toast + berries

Ten Family Lunch Menus

1. Sliced turkey + cheese + whole-grain crackers + carrot slices
2. Homemade pizza (whole-grain crust, tomato sauce, veggies, and cheese) + sliced pears

3. Chicken quesadilla + avocado chunks + peaches
4. Fruit/veggie smoothies + whole-grain crackers
5. Yogurt + sliced apples/berries + homemade whole-grain pita chips + baby carrots/green beans
6. Turkey/chicken burger or veggie burger + lettuce, tomato, cheese and a whole-grain bun + pineapple
7. Grilled cheese on whole-grain bread + tomato soup + blueberries
8. Turkey (and cheese on whole-grain bread) sandwiches + cherry tomatoes
9. Tuna or chicken salad + whole-grain pita + sliced cucumbers
10. Leftovers + mixed berries

Ten Family Dinner Menus

1. Whole-grain pasta (wheat or quinoa) + marinara sauce + sunflower seeds + sliced mango + green peas
2. Roasted chicken + homemade sweet potato French fries + broccoli + cut-up pears
3. Meatloaf + green beans + mashed sweet potatoes + strawberries
4. Beef, turkey, chicken, or veggie tacos + melon pieces
5. Homemade fish sticks or salmon + roasted sweet potatoes + cubed apples
6. Homemade pizza (whole-grain crust, cheese, and/or chicken pieces) + watermelon cubes
7. Turkey burger with whole-grain bun + orange slices + lettuce and tomato

8. Lasagna or pasta bake (whole-grain pasta, cheese, and veggies) + salad
9. Vegetarian bean chili + cornbread + roasted broccoli
10. Pot roast + sweet potatoes + green beans + apple slices

Modifying the Family Meal for Young Children

As soon as your baby begins to handle thicker, lumpier textures and finger foods, start adapting the family meal for him too, rather than serving separate foods. Oh, yeah, this means that you need to start eating *meals*. New parents so often serve lovingly prepared purees to the baby, while the adults desperately shovel in whatever they can scrounge. We know it's hard to cook a meal when you have a needy baby with a two-minute attention span. We get it. Start very small, on occasions when you have the energy and time. Find creative solutions such as the following:

- Start slow-cooker meals early in the day.
- If friends or family members want to come over, enlist their help to hold and entertain the baby while you whip up a quick meal.
- Cook extra food on weekends or whenever you have an extra pair of hands around.
- Rely on super-quick options like a store-roasted chicken and steam-in-a-bag veggies.

When your child is around age one, you can generally cut or shred many family foods into tiny pieces right at the table. If your child needs a smoother texture, a mini–food processor can pulse the food smaller in seconds.

Family Meal Dos and Don'ts

- Do go slowly, as your time and energy permit.
- Do decide what to serve (starting when your child is around age one) based on what the *family* likes to eat, not just what the *child* likes.
- Do serve a variety of foods (four or five is perfect) at a meal so that your child has plenty to choose from.
- Do have "Kids' Choice" night when the kids are older so that they can choose too!
- Do keep it *simple*!
- Do have a reasonable expectation for your child to sit at the table. Most very young children will be ready to get down from the table after about fifteen minutes, and that's okay.
- Do experiment with an appetizer at the table: cut-up fruits and veggies!
- Don't worry that your child won't get enough food if you serve what the family wants for dinner, not just what *she* wants.
- Don't cook a different meal because your child refuses what you made.

Screen Time: Media and Meals Don't Mix

Screens are everywhere, from televisions to smartphones to tablets, and they can be great for communication, entertainment, and even education. But my experience has taught me that too much screen time makes eating healthily very difficult. Limiting screen time can help your child stay on the path to healthy living.

Excessive screen time has been implicated in childhood obesity as well. How and to what extent media contributes to childhood obesity is a complex issue. Consider the following:

- Watching screens is a sedentary activity.
- Screen time displaces more active playtime.
- Children see thousands of unhealthy food advertisements every year on TV.
- The content of many popular TV shows teaches children bad habits.
- Mindless snacking (sometimes of unhealthy food) often happens in front of screens.
- Screen time at night makes for a later bedtime and poorer sleep quality.

➢ Dr. Tanya's Tip: Screen Time

The following suggestions will help you regulate recreational screen time for your children (homework/schoolwork not included):

- **AGE UNDER TWO:** Avoid as much as possible
- **AGES TWO THROUGH FIVE:** Under an hour total daily
- **AGES SIX THROUGH ELEVEN:** Under an hour total on school days, one to two hours on weekends

Get together with your partner, spouse, and other caregivers and come up with a media use plan. If you agree on rules ahead of time, you'll be less likely to cave if your toddler is crying for your phone or your preschooler is hitting the TV to get it to turn on.

Which, if any, of these factors is responsible for causing unhealthy eating and obesity in children? Likely it's a combination of all of the above, although most experts agree that the biggest offender is all the unhealthy food advertisements your child is exposed to via media.[13]

Advertising is extremely effective at getting children to request more junk food, eat less nutritious food, and attempt to influence their parents' food purchases.

The good news is that the problem is simple to control. Less screen time, combined with higher-quality screen time, makes for a healthier-

Q&A: Solutions for Real Parent Questions

Family Meal Issues

Q: I'm really frustrated because whenever I make a meal, someone (or everyone) complains. I don't feel like I'm a very good cook. I wind up just giving my kids whatever they want, because they don't like the food I cook.

A: Cooking is an art and a skill that doesn't always come naturally. First, decide how many meals a week you're willing to cook *without* compromise—meaning there's no alternative beyond what's served. Pair a new dish with an old favorite—for example, if you're making a new fish dish, serve it with the mashed potatoes you know they enjoy.

On the cooking front, you have many options available. Check out our recipes in chapter 15. Whenever you make something new, remember that adage I mentioned before: "Number one is a trial run." The first time you make something, it's just a rough draft! It may take a few tries to get the taste and texture right. Look for videos on the Internet for cooking advice, take a cooking class, or try new cookbooks from the library.

Q: My kids always want a heavy-carb dinner like pasta, tortillas, potatoes, or bread, but I don't want to eat so many starchy carbs for dinner. Any ideas?

weight child. Especially with very small children around, food and electronics need to be separated. When it's meal- or snacktime, turn the TV off; turn the phone to silent; turn the tablets off.

Some parents intentionally keep the television on during mealtime because it distracts their children and allows them to eat more. I prefer to reverse this practice, because if you have to distract your child to get her to eat, perhaps she isn't really hungry. And eating in front of the screen doesn't allow your child to learn how to self-regulate feeding and enjoy the natural colors, smells, textures, and look of her food.

A: Yes! Serve foods family-style and allow each family member to adjust the meal as he or she prefers. Here are some great examples:

- TACOS. Offer cooked meat (or a meatless option such as vegetarian refried beans), lettuce, chopped tomato, grated cheese, avocado/guacamole, salsa, and taco shells or tortillas. Parents who don't want carbs can make theirs into a salad.
- WHOLE-GRAIN PASTA. Offer turkey (or other meat) meatballs in marinara with pasta and vegetables. Parents can have the protein and vegetables and skip the pasta if they want. Alternatively, occasionally replace traditional pasta with spaghetti squash or quinoa pasta.
- CHICKEN AND POTATOES. Try homemade chicken tenders (see recipe on page 296), offered with roasted "French fries" (see recipe on page 292) and a large salad. Parents can put their chicken on the salad.

The answer lies in offering a great balanced meal from which everyone can choose. Ideally, though, you would want to put *some* of the potato, bread, or pasta on your plate—and eat it—so that your kids learn that healthy eating (as modeled by their parents) includes grains and carbs.

I've shared why I believe family meals are important and how to keep them super and simple. Now it's up to you to plan a little and incorporate meals into your family's busy life. Starting early will help set the routine and pattern for healthy family meals as your children grow. As your kids experience events during the day (both positive and challenging), they will think to themselves, "I'll share this with Mommy and Daddy tonight at dinner." It's a special way to create and share great memories with your child.

Remember This

- Families who eat together have better communication, less obesity, a healthier diet, and fewer picky eaters.
- Family meals may vary depending on your schedule, but try to incorporate as many such meals as possible, whether breakfasts, lunches, or dinners.
- Make meals a media-free time—always!
- Simple meals are super!
- Use the meal ideas in this chapter and the recipes in the final chapter to easily incorporate the Eleven Foundation Foods into your family meals.

PART THREE

Dr. Tanya's Advice on Tricky Issues

8.

Food Allergies and Food Intolerance

Eating Safe and Smart

Even if your child doesn't have a food allergy, I'm sure you know a child who does. Before having a child over at my house to play, I always ask the parent, "Is your child allergic to any foods?" The number of children with food allergies has skyrocketed over the past ten years, and we don't know exactly why. Food allergies now affect approximately 8 percent of children. According to a study released in 2013 by the Centers for Disease Control and Prevention, food allergies among children increased approximately 50% between 1997 and 2011.[14]

Eight foods account for 90 percent of all food-induced allergic reactions. These eight foods are *milk, eggs, peanuts, tree nuts, soy, wheat, fish, and shellfish.* I call these the "Big Eight." Children with allergies to milk, eggs, wheat, and soy are more likely to outgrow their allergies than are those who are allergic to peanuts, tree nuts, fish, and shellfish; allergies to the latter four are more likely to be lifelong.

The pediatrician's (and allergist's) approach to the introduction of commonly allergenic foods in infants and young children has dramatically changed over the past five to ten years. It was previously recommended to wait to give highly allergenic foods (such as egg whites, shellfish, peanuts, and tree nuts) until after two or even three years of age, depending on the child's family history of allergies. However, multiple studies have since shown that waiting to introduce such foods to infants who show no sign of allergic disease (such as eczema) *does not* decrease the chance of developing food allergies. That's great news, especially since these foods all have important nutrients for young children.[15]

So you don't *have* to wait to introduce allergenic foods, but when *should* you introduce them? Could feeding a baby such foods at a younger age actually *decrease* the development of food allergies?

Over the past year, everything we thought we knew about food allergies has been turned upside down. A recent landmark study showed that early introduction of peanut protein to high-risk infants actually *decreased* the chance of developing a peanut allergy![16] In this LEAP study (Learning Early About Peanut Allergy), researchers took around six hundred high-risk infants (those with evidence of eczema or egg allergies) who had tested negative or mildly allergic to peanuts by skin test at age four to eleven months. Half of each group ate peanut protein three times a week, and half avoided peanuts. At five years of age, of the infants who had initially tested negative, 14 percent of those in the group who avoided peanuts developed a peanut allergy, compared with 2 percent in the group who ate peanuts. That's a sevenfold difference! Of the infants who initially had a mildly positive skin test, 35 percent of those in the group who avoided peanuts got peanut allergies, compared with 11 percent in the group who received peanuts.

Basically, this study found that exposing infants to peanut protein three times a week dramatically reduced the incidence of peanut allergy. Wow! That's incredible data. The LEAP study convinced me to start making peanut butter oatmeal for my six-month-old, using approximately the amount of peanut protein given in the study. I'm now feeding it to him three times a week, and he loves it! (See our recipe for Peanut Butter Oatmeal on page 276.)

Additional studies are currently looking at very early introduction of other allergenic foods to see whether this decreases food allergies by allowing the body to develop tolerance to foods at an early stage.

So what does this mean for you as a parent? Pediatricians (and even allergists) don't have all the answers yet, but I recommend introducing healthy foods around six months of age in a consistency that your infant can handle, including some foods, like nut butters, eggs, and fish, that were previously discouraged due to their potential allergenic properties. Watch closely and make sure your child tolerates each food, and advance foods and consistencies as you feel your infant is ready. If your family has a history of food allergies, asthma, environmental allergies, or eczema, check with your pediatrician or allergist before starting your infant on the Big Eight.

When and How to Introduce the Big Eight

Current recommendations are that any foods (except honey) can be given to a child around six months of age. I like to introduce healthy foods early and often—as long as an infant doesn't have a reaction, of course. This includes the Big Eight, which again are milk (offer only yogurt and cheese under one year), eggs, peanuts, tree nuts, soy, wheat, fish, and shellfish.

If your child doesn't show any signs of allergies (see the section titled "Signs of a Food Allergy," below), you can introduce any of the Big Eight around six months of age as long as you serve them in the consistency, texture, and tiny size appropriate for your infant to eat. Although there needs to be more scientific research on the ideal time to introduce such foods, here is a list of my approximate ages for introducing potentially allergenic foods to your infant's diet:

- SIX TO EIGHT MONTHS: Dairy yogurt, peanut butter diluted to a nonsticky consistency (such as in oatmeal or a puffed snack food like Bamba), low-mercury fish (such as salmon), wheat (such as cereal)
- EIGHT TO NINE MONTHS: Eggs, peanut and almond butter on bread, shellfish (such as shrimp), soy products such as soft-cooked edamame
- ONE YEAR: Whole or 2 percent milk

Signs of a Food Allergy

Parents often ask me, "How do I know if my child has a food allergy?" Some signs of a food allergy are mild, such as a rash, while others are more severe, such as trouble breathing. As you introduce new foods to your child's diet, keep an eye out for signs of a food allergy.

Mild signs include eczema (a dry, scaly rash) and localized hives (a blotchy skin rash). Call your pediatrician for advice.

Severe signs include full-body hives, facial swelling, trouble breathing, and anaphylaxis (a life-threatening allergic reaction). If your child experiences any of these severe symptoms, call 911 immediately.

If you suspect that your child has a food allergy and you schedule an appointment to see your pediatrician, do a little prep work. Keep a log of specific symptoms and what your child had to eat or drink within two

Safety Tip

When to Call Your Pediatrician for Food Allergies: If your child has any allergic reaction, such as hives, vomiting, or lip swelling within two hours of eating any food, or gets a dry, itchy rash (eczema) within a few hours or days after eating a new food, stop the food and see your pediatrician right away.

hours before each symptom started. For older infants and children who may be eating foods with multiple ingredients or eating packaged foods, take a photo of the food label and take it, along with your symptom log, to your doctor's appointment.

Sometimes food allergies are obvious, such as, "My child ate a peanut and immediately developed hives." Other times it can take some detective work: "Each time my child eats a food baked with eggs and milk (such as a muffin or a cake), he gets a dry, itchy rash." Determining whether it was the eggs or the milk at fault is where the detective work comes in.

Once the culprit has been identified, your pediatrician or allergist may recommend strict avoidance of a food item (such as complete avoidance of milk) or only partial avoidance of the item (such as continuing to eat baked products made with milk). That decision will be based largely on the severity of the symptoms.

It's important to know, and to remember, that *food allergies can be life-threatening.* Some children are so allergic that eating a tiny piece of one peanut could kill them, while others may just develop eczema. If you have a child with food allergies, you must let everyone in her life know. This includes family members, caregivers, teachers, coaches, friends' parents, and anyone else who watches your child. In cases of a severe nut allergy, it may be recommended that you keep a nut-free home, to ensure that your child doesn't accidentally eat a nut. Some kids also wear a MedicAlert bracelet to alert anyone and everyone of their serious food allergy.

Identifying and Dealing with Food Allergies

If your child has a food reaction, your pediatrician may refer you to an allergist for further testing, such as lab work or skin testing to identify the specific food that caused the reaction. Allergy testing can be very helpful in determining which foods to avoid, which foods to serve, and how to treat future reactions.

Unfortunately, there is no cure for food allergies at this time. The only way to prevent reactions is to avoid your child's known food allergens. Unfortunately, accidental ingestions do occur.

If your child has a food allergy, you will become familiar with certain medications that you must carry everywhere and give to your child's daycare, school, family, friends, and neighbors. Ask your doctor for a written action plan so that you know which medications to use, how and when to use them, and how to call for help (such as when to call your pediatrician and when to call 911). Some common medications on action plans include:

EPINEPHRINE (generally administered by auto-injectable pen), which can be given for more severe symptoms, such as throat swelling, breathing difficulty, and anaphylaxis. It can also be given immediately after an accidental exposure—that is, even before symptoms—in the case of highly allergic individuals.

ANTIHISTAMINES (such as diphenhydramine), which can be given for an itchy mouth and eczema.

BRONCHODILATORS (such as albuterol, generally administered by inhaler), which can be given for coughing or wheezing.

Safety Tip

Severe Allergic Reactions: Do *not* rely on antihistamines and inhalers to treat a severe allergic reaction. The medication needed in that case is an injection of epinephrine. Let your doctor know immediately if your child is having a serious allergic reaction. Call 911 if your child is having trouble breathing or looks really sick, has full-body hives, has facial swelling, or is experiencing anaphylaxis.

Milk and Egg Allergies

You may be surprised to learn that approximately 75 percent of kids with milk or egg allergies, according to researchers, are able to eat baked products made with milk or eggs—things like muffins, waffles, or cake. The theory is that baking the food "denatures" the protein (a process that changes the structure of its amino acids), allowing the body to tolerate small amounts of the allergenic food. In addition, research shows that children who can tolerate baked milk or egg, and continue eating or being exposed to small amounts regularly, may have a higher chance of outgrowing their milk or egg allergy.[17]

How do you know if your allergic child can tolerate *baked* milk or egg? Ask your allergist if a baked milk or egg challenge is safe to be performed in the doctor's office under close observation. Do *not* try this at home, as some children will have a severe allergic reaction.

If your child passes the baked milk or egg challenge, your physician may instruct you to feed your child a product made with eggs or milk daily to allow your child's body to become tolerant to baked products made with those allergens.

If you're cooking at home, there are plenty of baked milk and egg pancake, waffle, and muffin recipes available, but always check with your allergist before giving such foods to your child.

Food Intolerance vs. Food Allergy

Food intolerance or sensitivity and food allergy can have similar symptoms, but it's important to know that they are *not* the same thing. A common example is lactose intolerance, which is not the same as a milk allergy.

True food allergies trigger an allergic immune system reaction in your body (a reaction that is IgE-mediated), which causes symptoms such as hives and trouble breathing, as noted earlier. True food allergies can be life-threatening.

Food intolerance or sensitivity, on the other hand, is not IgE-mediated, which means it is not an allergic reaction. With food intolerance or sensitivity, either the body cannot properly digest a specific food (such as dairy products containing lactose), or the digestive system is irritated by a specific substance (such as gluten, a form of protein found in certain grains). Symptoms of food intolerance can include nausea, gas, cramps, abdominal pain, diarrhea, irritability, nervousness, and headache.

Food intolerance symptoms generally come on gradually, and in some cases your child may be able to eat very small amounts of the offending food without trouble. You may also be able to take steps that help prevent a reaction. For example, if she has lactose intolerance, she may be able to drink lactose-free milk or take lactase enzyme pills that aid digestion.

Always talk to your pediatrician if your baby or child seems sensitive to a specific food. You do not want to remove foods without very good reason—especially entire categories of food (such as wheat). After evaluation and possible allergy testing, your pediatrician may refer you to a pediatric dietitian to ensure that your child gets proper nutrition if you need to remove an offending food or beverage from your child's diet.

Substitutions for Common Allergenic Foods

The good news when it comes to food allergies is that the 2006 Food Allergen Labeling and Consumer Protection Act requires companies to label foods in plain language if they contain the Big Eight. Companies can either list "Contains wheat" or "Contains nuts" (or whichever allergen applies), or list the food simply in the ingredient list—they can't just say "albumin," but instead must say "albumin (egg)." These labeling requirements make it easier for people to identify allergens in food. The bad news is that milk, soy, eggs, and wheat are in thousands of foods at the grocery store. So parents really need to take the time to carefully read labels and learn how to cook at home. Here are some common substitutions for allergenic foods to help you safely feed your child.

Wheat or Gluten

Your child may be allergic to wheat specifically (an allergic immune system reaction ideally confirmed by an allergist) or have celiac disease (a chronic immune-mediated disorder confirmed by a gastroenterologist—see below for more details). Most children allergic to wheat can eat other grains, such as barley, rye, and oats. However, people with celiac disease can't eat wheat, barley, rye, and some oats (oats are naturally gluten-free but can be cross-contaminated). The following meal suggestions address *both* wheat allergy and celiac disease:

- For breakfast, options include eggs with potatoes, gluten-free bread for toast or French toast, rice- or corn-based cold cereal, hot oatmeal, oatmeal muffins, commercial gluten-free waffles, and breakfast burritos made with corn tortillas.
- For dinner, serve brown rice, potatoes, sweet potatoes, beans, lentils, quinoa, polenta, and corn tortillas.
- Great snack or lunch ideas can include yogurt, cheese, nuts or nut butters, sliced turkey, tuna or egg or chicken salad, popcorn, and a quesadilla made with a corn tortilla.

Eggs

If your child has an egg allergy, work closely with your allergist to determine whether the child can tolerate eggs in baked products, or if he must avoid *all* products made with any egg (see above for an explanation). Here are some suggestions for meal and snack alternatives that don't contain egg:

- For breakfast, serve turkey bacon or turkey sausage; whole-grain, low-sugar cereal with milk is another great option, along with nuts or nut butter on toast.
- Try cake recipes from vegan cookbooks. You'll find lots of tips for egg substitutes. One popular substitution for 1 whole egg is flaxseed plus water—mix 1 tablespoon flaxseed meal with 3 tablespoons water and let the mixture sit for five minutes before proceeding.
- When making meatloaf or meatballs, you can usually omit the egg with good results.
- In a cookie or other baked good, try substituting a half banana or ¼ cup applesauce per egg. Natural-food stores also commonly carry commercial egg replacement products. The texture will change, but it can be acceptable in items such as banana bread or cookies.
- Try a yogurt smoothie for breakfast or snack.

Soy

Most individuals allergic to soy can safely eat soy lecithin and soy oils, which allows them to eat the many foods that contain these ingredients. Studies show that most allergic individuals can safely eat soy oil that has been highly refined (though they should still avoid cold-pressed, expeller-pressed, or extruded soybean oil). In fact, the FDA exempts highly refined soybean oil from being labeled as an allergen. If you have any questions, ask your allergist.

- Avoid most commercial veggie burgers and meatless sausage, bacon, and other meat.
- The longer the ingredient list on a processed food, the more likely it will contain something derived from soy, so make sure you read

the label carefully. Look for products with shorter ingredient lists, instead.

- Many products touted as "high-protein," such as protein-added cereals, granola bars, and baked goods, contain soy. For example, while the high-protein variety of a popular "O" cereal has soy, the original version does not contain any soy.

Milk/Dairy

Work closely with your allergist and pediatrician, because some kids need to avoid all dairy—including yogurt and cheese—while others may need to avoid only liquid milk.

- Read the section on milk and egg allergies (above) and speak with your allergist or pediatrician about including products with cooked or baked dairy.
- Of the various milk alternatives, soy milk is the substitute closest to dairy milk in calories and protein.
- Almond, rice, and coconut milk are all low in protein. If your family drinks these items, you must include protein in other forms, such as eggs, red meat, chicken, fish, and nuts, to ensure that your growing child gets enough protein.
- Take advantage of vegan and kosher meat or kosher pareve recipes, which will not include any dairy.

Peanuts

Nut allergies can be life-threatening, so in many cases strict avoidance (along with carrying an epinephrine auto-injector pen twenty-four/seven) is your best option. Here are some nut-free options that your child can enjoy:

- Sunflower-seed butter is a great alternative for kids allergic to both peanut and tree nuts. No-nut butters made from a variety of foods (including golden peas) are available. I've tried them, and they're delicious!
- If your child is allergic only to peanuts, but is able to eat tree nuts without any reaction, then almond butter is a healthy and tasty option. Other tree-nut butters, such as cashew and hazelnut butters, are also peanut-free options. If you're unsure which nuts your child is allergic to, double-check with your allergist or pediatrician.
- Join a peanut allergy group online for support, recipes, and meal ideas.

Celiac Disease

Unlike a wheat allergy or simple gluten intolerance, celiac disease is an autoimmune disorder in which gluten, the protein found in wheat, rye, and barley (and foods derived from those grains) triggers a severe physiological response. In children with celiac disease, gluten damages the part of the intestines responsible for absorbing nutrients from food. When that happens, they can't absorb needed nutrients properly and can become malnourished. Infants may fail to gain weight and grow; older kids may have diarrhea, abdominal pain, bloating, weight loss, and fatigue.

Celiac disease tends to run in families, so if you have a family history of celiac disease, your child may have a higher risk of developing it. If you're concerned that your child may have celiac disease, talk to your pediatrician about testing and/or referral to a pediatric gastroenterologist.

Celiac disease is treated by not eating gluten. Avoiding gluten can be difficult, because it's found in many foods, but a dietitian can help you with a diet plan to ensure that your child gets proper nutrition for growth and development while avoiding gluten.

Parents of a child with celiac disease now have a much different experience at the grocery store than did parents in the years before the explosive gluten-free trend. Celiac patients have definitely benefited from the thousands of gluten-free products now available, including pretzels, breads, cereals, granola bars, tortillas, and even pizza and pasta. The benefits are ease and convenience and the assurance of a gluten-free product, but good nutrition doesn't always result.

➢ Dr. Tanya's Tip: Food-Allergic Kids

At Home

Consider keeping your house or a section of your kitchen, fridge, or pantry "allergy-free," depending on what foods your child is allergic to. If you have children who are allergic to different items, label *everything* to avoid cross-contamination or accidental ingestion of an allergenic food. Vegan cookbooks can provide many great, creative recipes for kids allergic to eggs or dairy.

At School

Give the teacher a bag of store-bought, individually wrapped treats that are safe for your child to eat. When there is an impromptu party or special event where food is brought to class, the teacher can offer your child a safe treat from your stash. If possible, volunteer to bring a food item to a class party that you know is safe for your child and others with food allergies to eat.

At Restaurants

Talk to the wait staff or chef about your child's food allergies. Many restaurants are understanding and accommodating. That said, even "safe foods" may accidentally have cross-contamination with something your child is allergic to (from a cooking pan or utensils). If your child has life-threatening allergies, ask if a separate pan and utensils can be used, instead of a griddle where other foods have been prepared.

BETH'S GROCERY GUIDE

Healthy Gluten-Free Options

Before packing your pantry with gluten-free *processed* foods, stock up on these healthy gluten-free items with either one ingredient or a very short ingredient list (always check food labels to ensure that the item is truly gluten-free):

- All fruit
- All vegetables (potatoes and sweet potatoes can be used as a starch instead of bread or pasta; you can roast, mash, or bake them)
- Rolled oats (oats are naturally gluten-free but can be cross-contaminated, so to be safe choose gluten-free oats)
- Rice
- Nuts and seeds
- Eggs
- Fish, chicken, meat
- Edamame
- Beans and lentils
- Corn tortillas
- Nut or seed butters such as peanut butter, almond butter, and sesame-seed butter
- Dairy products such as milk, yogurt, and cheese

The Gluten-Free Family Meal

Since a gluten-free child is often eating different foods than his fellow students, family, and friends, we think it's valuable to have at least a few gluten-free meals per week that *everyone* in the family can enjoy. Sitting down to the same meal together is good for preventing pickiness, encouraging inclusion, and creating a happy, relaxed mealtime experience. Some easy and inclusive meals are listed below:

- Chicken or beef tacos made with spices or a gluten-free seasoning packet, served alongside toppings such as veggies, guacamole, sour cream, cheese, and salsa, with corn tortillas (perhaps both hard taco shells and warmed soft tortillas)
- Barbecued chicken (with gluten-free barbecue sauce), along with rice or roasted potatoes, green beans, and melon cubes
- Steak with sweet potato fries and sliced apples
- Meatballs and marinara over gluten-free pasta (such as quinoa pasta)
- Quesadillas made with corn tortillas, black beans, and bell peppers
- Omelet or scrambled eggs with lean bacon or turkey bacon and fruit
- Beans with rice, along with a salad
- Lentil soup and gluten-free cornbread
- Gluten-free cereal with milk, topped with fruit
- Chicken drumsticks, corn on the cob, and fruit
- Almond-Oat Granola Bars (see recipe on page 301), milk, and fruit

Overall, it's best to save gluten-free processed foods for occasions when you really need the ease and convenience, rather than relying on them for everyday staples. A gluten-free pretzel or granola bar is fine for an occasional snack or to send to school for lunch or a party, but too many highly processed gluten-free products crowd out the many naturally healthy gluten-free options that are available.

As we've seen, recommendations on feeding children the Big Eight have changed dramatically over the past few years, with new guidelines stating that allergenic foods such as milk (before age one, give only yogurt and cheese), eggs, peanuts, tree nuts, soy, wheat, fish, and shellfish can be introduced around six months of age in a consistency that a baby can handle, as long as they're well tolerated. Promising research has shown that early introduction of peanut protein, followed by frequent exposure to it, may decrease the chance of a child's becoming allergic later in life. Only time (and more research) will show whether this applies to the other allergenic foods as well. As a parent as well as a pediatrician, I suggest early introduction and frequent feeding of all Eleven Foundation Foods, including the Big Eight, with close observation for signs of allergic reaction.

Remember This

- It's okay to start allergenic foods (the Big Eight) around six months of age in a consistency that your baby can handle.
- If your egg- or milk-allergic child can tolerate baked egg or milk (without an allergic reaction), keep offering it.
- Call your pediatrician immediately if your child has an allergic reaction such as hives, vomiting, or lip swelling within two hours of eating any food. If your child gets a dry, itchy rash (eczema) within a few hours or days after eating a new food, stop the food and see your pediatrician right away.
- If your child must avoid a certain food due to an allergy, make sure she gets proper nutrition through other foods. Consult a dietitian if needed.
- Send a bag of safe snacks/treats to school for your child to have during special class parties and events.
- If your child has a food allergy, see your allergist every year to determine when and if it is safe to try to introduce the allergenic food to your child's diet.

9.

Sugar

The Good, the Bad, and the Really Ugly

Sugar. It makes food taste so good, and once little taste buds try it, they're usually hooked. Now, sugar isn't *all* bad, and it certainly has a place in your child's diet, but not the *prime* place! Unfortunately, most of us—kids and adults alike—consume far too much added sugar, which displaces healthy foods and can create many feeding, eating, and health problems.

Added sugar is a problem because it has infiltrated almost every processed food and because it's so commonplace and inexpensive. I counted fifty-seven different candy bars in one checkout line of my local store!

Sugar is a treat and should be treated as such. Don't worry as much about sugar you add yourself to things you make at home—in muffins and homemade desserts, for example. You have control over these items. Worry more about how much sugar is added by companies to seemingly innocent foods such as oatmeal and granola bars.

In this chapter we will answer the many questions parents have about sugar, and develop a game plan to help you make sweet and smart choices.

Five Sweet Steps

Let's start at the grocery store, where most confusion occurs. Picture the grocery store as your very own real-life Candy Land game. Here are five rules that help parents navigate through the aisles. I call them Sweet Steps:

1. Remember that sugar is for treats.
2. Add your own sugar (if needed).
3. Buy food with a short ingredient list. Remember: *Five or less is best; more than ten, think again.*
4. Avoid food with fake colors.
5. Join the "one" club.

Let's look at each of these Sweet Steps in turn.

Sweet Step 1: Remember That Sugar Is for Treats

Candy Land is honest. Peppermint Forest, Lollipop Woods, and Chocolate Swamp sound like what they are: sweet treats. Imagine a new version of Candy Land with the following highlights: Syrupy Yogurt Springs, Gummy Gushers, and Monster Muffins. Unlike the Peppermint Forest, these we can find in the aisles of our grocery stores!

It's best to try to limit sugary foods (parents, this is for you too!) to the dessert/treat category, instead of having them infiltrate breakfast, lunch, dinner, and snacks. Here are some common sources of *hidden* sugar at the grocery store:

- Flavored oatmeal
- Fruit-flavored yogurt and yogurt with toppings

- Muffins and scones
- Fruit gummies
- Granola bars, fruit bars, and snack bars
- Cereals
- Frozen waffles, French toast sticks, pancakes, toaster pastries
- Toddler specialty products
- Kid-specific lunch packs
- Sports drinks, juices, and lemonade

Everyone knows that ice cream and candy are sweet treats. But when you give your child flavored oatmeal in the morning, fruit gummies at snack, and a premade pack at lunch, you're pushing sources of sugar all day long, which is not healthy for anyone, particularly a growing and developing child.

Sugar is for treats, *not* for regular foods. Maybe you're thinking about your pantry and starting to feel guilty about all the sugary treats lurking there. Stop! Let go of guilt and instead give your pantry and your household what I call a "sugar makeover." In no time, you'll be on your way to creating better habits around buying and consuming sugar for your family.

Conducting a sugar makeover. Giving your household a sugar makeover can really make a difference in cutting down on excess hidden sugar—especially when it comes to foods that don't need added sugar. Remember: a child's nutritional habits follow the parents' example. As hard as it can be to give up those sugary coffee drinks, doing so goes a long way in modeling good habits for your child. Over the next few pages I'll share two examples of a sugar makeover, one for adults and one for children, showing daily sugar intake both before and after. First, though, to provide context, here are the recommended daily added

Q&A: Solutions for Real Parent Questions

The Dessert Dilemma

Q: My child wants treats all day. What do I do?

A: There are many "right" answers to the dessert dilemma. I've seen extreme sugar restriction to extreme permissiveness. Sometimes extremely permissive parents weren't allowed to have any sweets as a child or vice versa. As with most things, a middle approach tends to be best. Try one of these three strategies:

1. Offer fruit for dessert on weeknights and a small treat on weekends.
2. Give a small treat no more than once a day if your child is asking for one and if you feel comfortable giving it. Beth uses tiny serving dishes to teach her daughter the right portion size for dessert—look for small dishes you might use to serve a condiment.
3. Don't adopt a strict "policy"; just emphasize small portions of treats, with frequency depending on the day and situation.

Whatever treat strategy you choose, try to keep the following guidelines in mind to reduce excess and hidden sugars:

- SHOP. Buy food with short ingredient lists (or one-ingredient foods such as fruit).
- TEACH. Explain to your child that "sugar is a treat."
- BAKE. When you bake, make mini-sizes—mini-muffins, mini-cookies with mini-chocolate chips
- DIP. Dip fruit into chocolate for dessert.
- MAKE YOUR OWN. Make your own 100 percent-juice popsicles.
- SERVE SMALL. Put ice cream and treats into small bowls, using small spoons. Have a monetary limit for the frozen yogurt shop, where portions can be huge due to big containers.

sugar limits (from the American Heart Association, Beth, and me)—that is, the maximum amount recommended, which means everyone should have less.

WOMEN: 6 teaspoons

MEN: 9 teaspoons

KIDS: 4 teaspoons or less, depending on age

1 teaspoon = 4 grams of sugar

Adult Sugar Intake "Before"

- Iced caramel coffee drink, reduced-fat muffin
- Regular 6-ounce low-fat yogurt
- Salad
- Chicken, rice, vegetable
- 2 cookies
- Estimated added teaspoons sugar: 21 (really bad)

Adult Sugar Intake "After"

- Unsweetened latte with 1 teaspoon sugar (added by *you*)
- Whole-wheat toast with peanut butter and thinly spread fruit preserve
- Whole-grain cracker or nuts
- Salad
- Chicken, rice, vegetable
- 2 small cookies
- Estimated added teaspoons sugar: 4 to 5 (much better)

Child Sugar Intake "Before"

- 2 chocolate-chip frozen waffles
- Graham crackers
- Fruit gummy pack, yogurt with colored cereal topping, carrots
- String cheese
- Small milkshake or frozen yogurt
- Chicken, rice, vegetable
- 5 small chocolate pieces
- Estimated added teaspoons sugar: 11 (really bad)

BETH'S GROCERY GUIDE

Sugar on Product Labels

Under current regulations, "sugar" is listed by grams on food labels. There is no differentiation between "natural" and "added" sugars. The most common natural sugars are those found in fruit and dairy products. These natural sugars—fructose and lactose—are part of a normal, healthy diet. If you look on the ingredient list, you won't see any *added* sugar listed for fruit or (unsugared) dairy products. In fact, a medium apple has 19 grams of sugar, but you don't have to worry about that kind of sugar. Apples don't even need a food label, because all the sugar is naturally occurring. Regulations may soon (I hope) change to require manufacturers to list "added" sugars separately from "natural" sugars. What a help that will be! Until then, look at the ingredient list to determine whether a product has sugar added.

Let's look at milk. One cup of milk equals 13 grams of "natural" (not added) sugar, or about 3 teaspoons. This is naturally occurring sugar, remember—nothing that a food company has added—and therefore it's completely fine. A cup of chocolate milk has 26 grams of sugar, but

Child Sugar Intake "After"

- 2 whole-grain waffles with 1 teaspoon real maple syrup
- Dry "O" cereal
- Regular 4-ounce yogurt (no fake colors), carrots, apple
- String cheese
- Water, fruit, turkey slice, whole-grain crackers after school
- Chicken, rice, vegetable
- 2 small chocolate pieces
- Estimated added teaspoons sugar: 4½ (much better)

---

the labeling doesn't differentiate between natural milk sugar (lactose) and added flavoring. So you have to subtract the natural sugar yourself, which leaves 13 grams of added sugar.

You might also have to convert the serving size so that you're comparing equal amounts. Here's an example of the math you would need to do to determine the grams of sugar added to two different yogurts:

> 8-ounce plain yogurt = 12 grams sugar (which means 3 grams lactose or naturally occurring sugar in every 2 ounces)
>
> 6-ounce low-fat flavored yogurt = 27 grams total sugar (which means 18 grams added sugar, or 4½ teaspoons added sugar)
>
> 4-ounce "kid" yogurt with fake-colored cereal topping = 13 grams total sugar (which means 7 grams added sugar, or almost 2 teaspoons added sugar)

Such time-consuming and confusing calculations are presently the only way to determine exactly how much added sugar is in a product. What sleep-deprived parent has the time for that?

Sweet Step 2:
Add Your Own Sugar (If Needed)

This Sweet Step deals mainly with sweetened drinks, which are often little more than liquid sugar. Let's look first at the drinks many adults favor.

Adults may not consider a vanilla latte, caramel macchiato, or lemonade a sugary treat, but these drinks often have more sugar than cookies or candy. Here are the teaspoons of added sugar in some popular sweetened coffee drinks:

Small caramel macchiato or vanilla latte = 4 teaspoons

Medium white-chocolate mocha = 9 teaspoons

Large java-chip iced coffee = 18½ teaspoons

Why subject your body to all that extra sugar when it's so easy to reduce your sugar from drinks? Simply order a plain latte or plain tea or coffee and sweeten it yourself. If you order flavoring, ask your barista to use half (or even less) of the usual amount of flavoring.

When it comes to kids, it's best to just not buy any drink with sugar added to it. If you buy juice boxes, select only 100 percent juice with no sugar added. Some stores also sell juice boxes that are half juice, half water, likewise a good option. If ordering juice out, ask for it to be diluted with half water. When ordering chocolate milk or hot chocolate out, ask if half the syrup can be used to decrease sugar. Hot chocolate made with milk is more nutritious than if it is made with water and a powdered mix.

The rise in our country's obesity rates directly correlates with the rise in sugar-sweetened drink consumption among both adults and children. That's because our bodies don't eat less to compensate for the calories consumed in soda or juice—they're just extra calories, which can mean extra weight.

All parents and kids should drink water instead of soda, juice, lemonade, heavily sweetened coffee, and sports drinks. Two of the healthiest things parents can do for their children are never buy sugar-sweetened drinks, and stop drinking sugar-sweetened beverages in front of them. Sugar-sweetened drinks are hardly ever appropriate for kids. Parents often don't realize how quickly these calories add up. Just one such drink twice a week—perhaps lemonade at lunch, and a regular soda on the weekend—can easily add up to 500 extra calories; and many kids consume these drinks far more frequently than that.

Simply put, water is the best thing for you and your children to drink regularly. It's a healthy habit that begins early and lasts a lifetime.

Note: Avoid the kid's meal trap—a drink included with a kid's entrée. Even if juice or soda is included with your purchase, don't serve it to your child. It's much healthier to order water or milk for her instead, even if you have to pay a bit extra for the milk.

BETH'S GROCERY GUIDE

Reduced-Sugar or No-Sugar-Added Products

Many "reduced-sugar" and "low-sugar" products have artificial sweeteners instead of sugar. I don't recommend these products for children, for a couple of reasons. A sip once in a while is okay for your child, but don't make it a regular habit. Not only are artificial sweeteners refined chemicals, but they also get children hooked on an extra-sweet taste. Watch out especially for oatmeal, ice cream, and yogurt with "lower sugar"; check these food labels for artificial sweeteners. You want to buy products that simply use less sugar, not that substitute other chemicals for an even sweeter taste.

It's quite possible that if stricter sugar labeling laws come down the pike, as expected—laws that require manufacturers to list added sugar separately—there will be a big increase in the use of artificial sweeteners, in order to keep the grams of added sugar down. Then it will be important to keep an eye out for, and try to avoid, artificial sugar as well.

Sweet Step 3: Buy Food with a Short Ingredient List

The longer a food's ingredient list, the more likely it will contain multiple sources of sugar. All of the following—whether organic or not, whether non-GMO or not—are sources of added sugar:

- Glucose
- Honey
- Fruit juice concentrate
- Sucrose
- Fructose
- High-fructose corn syrup
- Corn syrup
- Corn syrup solids
- Dextrose
- Molasses
- Fruit juice nectar
- Invert sugar
- Malt syrup
- Brown sugar in the raw
- Sugar-cane juice

So, should you run for the hills if you see any of these on your food label? Not necessarily. But do use caution, not only with added sugar but with added *anything*. You've already been introduced to my tricks for managing ingredient lists:

Five or less is best. This rule goes for any processed food, including cereal, crackers, bread, oatmeal, granola bars, chips, flavored coffee creamer, drinks, fruit snacks (such as gummies), protein bars, yogurt, and frozen foods. You don't have to include vitamins and minerals in your count, even if they're listed separately (as they are on cereal boxes). You'll be surprised at the number of sugar sources you find in reportedly or so-called "healthy" foods.

One-ingredient foods, including the Eleven Foundation Foods, are true winners: fruits, vegetables, beans, lentils, nuts, milk, eggs, chicken, fish, and so on. Do *not* worry about the sugar in one-ingredient foods. Ignore anyone who tells you that carrots, for example, are high in sugar. They're vegetables with naturally occurring sugar as well as important vitamins and nutrients, and they're *good* for you!

More than ten, think again. Once a food has over ten ingredients, the likelihood goes way up that it contains many added sugars. Best not to buy foods with more than ten ingredients, unless the ingredients are all things you would find in your own kitchen and you can pronounce everything on the label.

➢ Dr. Tanya's Tip: Don't Be a Carb Counter

Counting or limiting carbohydrates may be trendy for some adults, but it's not a good idea for kids. You don't want to raise children to be carb counters. Children with diabetes who need to count carbs to dose their insulin are, of course, an exception. In general, carbs (aka carbohydrates) are important for a growing child and are part of a balanced diet. That said, choose your carbs wisely. Whole-grain carbs are always a better choice, not only for nutrition, but to get your child used to the taste and look of whole grains from a young age. And the carbs found naturally in fruits and vegetables are not only totally fine, but important for a child's proper growth and development.

Sweet Step 4:
Avoid Food with Fake (aka Artificial) Colors

Food dyes make junky food appear exciting compared to real food. Compare brightly colored stretchy fruit rolls to plain fruit, for example. You can see why kids are drawn to the fake colors.

You'll know if a food contains a fake color if it includes an ingredient labeled as noted in this description, straight from the FDA:

> *Certified color additives have special names consisting of a prefix, such as FD&C, D&C, or Ext. D&C; a color; and a number. An example is FD&C Yellow No. 6, often found in cereals, ice cream, and baked goods. Sometimes a color additive is identified by a shortened form of its name, consisting of just the color and number, such as Yellow 6.*

When I explain food dyes to children, I tell them to check food labels for anything with a color and a number, and to avoid those products, because consuming food dyes is like adding paint to your food. Even beige foods, like some cereals and oatmeals, have artificial color added, though they might not look vibrantly colored. Check the ingredient list!

You might be wondering why this comes up here, in a discussion about sugar. It's because if a food has fake color, it also generally has added sugar (and other junk too!). Unfortunately, most food marketed specifically to kids contains fake colors. As a rule, stay away from such foods. (See more information about food dyes on page 208).

Sweet Step 5:
Join the "One" Club

One-ingredient foods may have natural sugar, but they have absolutely no added sugar, so these simple foods get a grade A! Recipes you make in your own kitchen, from scratch, are almost universally good choices, in large part because they result primarily from one-ingredient foods.

If you happen to make muffins or cookies or bread, freeze the extras; they're certainly healthier than what you would buy premade at the

BETH'S GROCERY GUIDE

Ketchup Kids

During an interview about the movie *Fed Up*, one of the producers mentioned ketchup as a sugar source. I looked at my ketchup label, and sure enough, it listed 4 grams of sugar per tablespoon-size serving—that's 1 teaspoon of sugar! Some brands may also have fake colors included on the ingredient list. My older child puts "ketchup on her ketchup," so I got a little concerned and decided to investigate. Here's what I found out:

- 1 tablespoon tomato paste has 2 grams sugar. This is naturally occurring from the dried tomato product—in other words, no sugar added.
- 1 tablespoon ketchup has 4 grams sugar. Combining this fact with the previous one, we're looking at about 2 grams naturally occurring sugar and about 2 grams added. In other words, for every 1 tablespoon of ketchup you eat, you're also getting just over ½ teaspoon added sugar.

As a result, I've switched our household to a "simple" ketchup—one with only one sugar ingredient and no corn syrup or fake colors. I've decided not to sweat a tablespoon of ketchup, especially if it's served along with healthy food I made in my own kitchen. If your child wants to dip her homemade veggies or chicken into "simple" ketchup at home, I'd say let her; I'd rather have her eat the home-cooked veggies and chicken with a little ketchup than not eat them at all.

➢ Dr. Tanya's Tip: Food Label Detectives

Once your kids can read, teach them to identify fake colors on a label. It's a fun game and a good lesson for choosing healthier food options over junky ones.

store. You'll often hear nutritionists suggest shopping the perimeter of the store instead of the inner aisles. That's because most healthy foods reside around the edges (dairy, produce, meat, and so on). The simplest choice you can make: one is the best number.

Sugar is a part of every diet, but we do need to understand that it's a treat and should be treated as such. Remember: don't worry as much about foods you cook at home and sweeten yourself. Worry instead about how much sugar was added before you bought a commercially made product. If your grocery cart is full of foods targeted to children, chances are your child's sugar intake will far exceed what is okay for his small body. Follow the five Sweet Steps to making your family healthier!

Remember This

- Buy one-ingredient foods whenever possible.
- Read labels and look for shorter ingredient lists. Count ingredients before making any food purchase. *Five or less is best; more than ten, think again!*
- Don't worry about naturally occurring sugar, such as that in fruit, milk, and unsweetened dairy products; it's fine.
- Avoid fake colors, especially in cereal and snack products.
- Remember that added sugar is for treats, not to dominate the day's meals and snacks. Give your household a sugar makeover, to keep sugary treats to a healthy amount.

10.

Vegetarian and Vegan Kids

Planting the Seeds of Growth

In the early 1970s, Kermit the Frog famously sang, "It's not easy being green." Families who want to go green today have a much easier experience than Kermit did! Vegetarian and vegan adults can choose from hundreds of amazing cookbooks and food blogs for help cooking anything from the simplest appetizer to a full-on dinner party. There are now tons of restaurant and grocery store options to make eating a plant-based diet more convenient. But kids are not little adults! You have to be a little more zealous and take a little more care raising a young child on a vegetarian or vegan diet, to be sure he is getting proper nutrition.

It is completely possible to raise a healthy vegetarian or vegan child as long as you educate yourself about proper nutrition and ensure that your child is getting enough of all the nutrients needed to grow and develop. This chapter sets out what you need to know to guard your child from nutritional deficiencies and provide the best possible nutrition you can on a green diet.

Raising Children on a Vegetarian Diet

I will discuss vegetarian issues first and then move on to raising a vegan child.

Protein in a Vegetarian Diet

Protein is necessary for growth, and birth to age five is a critical growth period for children. Give your vegetarian child varied sources of protein so that she receives a good balance of amino acids. Vegetarian sources of protein include:

- Eggs
- Dairy (milk, yogurt, cheese, cottage cheese)
- Beans and lentils
- Soy milk, edamame, and tofu
- Nuts and nut butters
- Fish (for pescetarians—that is, vegetarians who also eat fish)

Dairy, eggs, and soy all offer "complete" proteins, meaning proteins that have the full complement of essential amino acids. When it comes to some nonanimal protein sources (like beans and nuts), combining multiple sources throughout the day ensures better absorption of amino acids. (See the vegan section later in the chapter for a further explanation.) If you offer your vegetarian child protein-rich foods three times a day in age-appropriate portions, he will generally get the grams of protein needed for proper growth.

Iron in a Vegetarian Diet

Since vegetarian children don't eat meat, it's critical that you focus on their consumption of iron-rich foods. Infants and toddlers who don't

➢ Dr. Tanya's Tip: Soy Got a Bad Rap

Some parents tell me that they don't want to include soy in the family diet because they've heard it speeds up the onset of puberty in children (particularly girls) by increasing their estrogen levels. Soy contains *plant* estrogens, not human estrogens; and although plant estrogens do bind to human estrogen receptors, they have a very weak effect. Rest assured, soy from natural sources (such as tofu, edamame, and soy milk) is a healthy source of protein and is *not* a cause of early puberty. In fact, natural soy may actually protect girls from developing prematurely, and in some cases may delay puberty.[18] This may not hold true, however, for manufactured soy products (like soy protein isolate) found in many foods, such as protein bars. Again, one-ingredient, natural foods are healthier.

receive enough iron can have poor mental and physical growth and development.

Vegetarian sources of iron include:

- Eggs (especially egg yolks)
- Iron-fortified cereals (especially baby cereals and raisin brans)
- Whole grains
- Beans, lentils, and other legumes
- Dried fruit (such as prunes, raisins, apricots)
- Broccoli, spinach, kale, collards, asparagus
- Blackstrap molasses
- Salmon/tuna (if you eat fish)

Cooking Help Desk

Increasing Iron Absorption: Iron from vegetables, fruits, and grains, called nonheme iron, is less available for absorption than the heme iron found in meat, fish, and poultry. If you want to increase absorption of both types of iron, serve iron-rich foods with foods high in vitamin C, such as oranges, orange juice, other citrus fruits, bell peppers, tomatoes, or tomato sauce. You could, for example, serve scrambled eggs with orange slices, or beans and rice in a tomato sauce. Another trick to increase iron is cooking in a cast-iron pan. The food will absorb a little bit of the iron from the pan.

Vitamin B_{12} and Zinc in a Vegetarian Diet

Vitamin B_{12} helps the body make DNA, is essential for healthy nerve and blood cells, and helps prevent a certain type of anemia. Since vitamin B_{12} is found mainly in animal products, a vegan diet and some vegetarian diets will need vitamin B_{12} supplements under the guidance of a physician. Vegetarian sources of vitamin B_{12} include cheese and eggs. Many grain products (especially cereals) are also fortified with vitamin

➢ Dr. Tanya's Tip: A Daily Multivitamin

Although food is the best source of vitamins, a good way to ensure that your vegetarian or vegan child gets enough zinc, vitamin B_{12}, calcium, vitamin D, and iron every day is to give a daily children's multivitamin that contains each of those nutrients. What type of vitamin is best? The one that your kids like taking every day! A vitamin in your pantry that your kids refuse to take doesn't help anyone. Remember to store all vitamins up high, out of a child's reach.

B_{12}. Plant foods do not usually contain vitamin B_{12} unless they are fortified. Speak with your pediatrician about your child's diet and the possible need to supplement with vitamin B_{12}.

Some vegetarian diets may also be low in zinc, a mineral that helps the human immune system function properly and is needed to activate many pathways in the body. About half the dietary zinc consumed in the United States comes from animal products, especially beef. Vegetarian sources of zinc include milk products, beans, and fortified cereals. Talk to your pediatrician about whether your child would benefit from a zinc supplement.

Family-Friendly Vegetarian Meal Ideas

Items from the Eleven Foundation Foods are well represented in the list below. Feel free to add any fruit or vegetable your family likes to these suggested meals.

Breakfast Ideas

- Scrambled egg, whole-wheat toast, orange slices
- French toast
- Whole-wheat frozen or homemade waffle spread with nut butter or with a side of cottage cheese
- Yogurt, fruit, whole-grain cereal
- Whole-grain pancakes with a side of cottage cheese or yogurt
- Avocado and vegetables on toast
- Whole-grain toast with scrambled egg, or "egg in a hole" (directions: in a skillet, toast bread with a hole cut in the middle; then crack an egg into the center and cook it)
- Whole-grain cereal with milk and fruit

Lunch or Dinner Ideas

- Nut butter sandwich (whole-grain bread, almond or peanut butter, and jam or mashed fruit), side of fruit or vegetables
- Grilled cheese (on whole-grain bread), sliced pears
- Whole-grain pasta, fruit, sunflower seeds or nuts
- Burrito made with vegetarian refried beans and cheese
- Chili made with ground tofu-based "meat," beans, a sprinkle of shredded cheese
- Vegetarian lasagna
- Cheese and vegetable pizza
- Whole-grain English muffin or bagel pizzas (with pizza sauce, cheese, and vegetables)
- Cheese cubes, fruit, roasted "French fries" (see recipe on page 292)
- Lentil soup (see recipe on page 295) with cornbread
- Macaroni and cheese (made with whole-grain or quinoa pasta and vegetables, see recipe on page 286)
- Sweet potato (roasted, mashed, or baked as "fries") with edamame
- Potato pancakes with sour cream and applesauce (for dipping)

Safety Tip

When to Call Your Pediatrician About a Vegetarian Diet: Overall, it's a good idea to communicate with your pediatrician about your family's vegetarian diet. If any issues arise with growth or nutrient deficiencies, there are many options available to ensure that your child gets the nutrients needed to grow and develop properly.

- Avocado and vegetable sandwich
- Whole-grain pita pocket stuffed with hummus and veggies
- Cheesy rice or quinoa with broccoli
- Canned beans, cooked rice, shredded cheese

Snack Ideas

- Smoothie made with yogurt, frozen peaches, or berries (see Berry Smoothie recipe on page 303)
- Smoothie made with milk, nut butter, and a small squeeze of chocolate syrup if desired (see Super Smoothie recipe on page 304)
- Edamame and whole-grain pita chips
- Hummus and pretzel thins
- Avocado (as guacamole) with organic white corn chips or whole-grain pita chips (see recipe on page 307)
- Whole-grain crackers spread with cheese, cream cheese, cottage cheese, or Greek yogurt
- Graham cracker with almond or peanut butter
- Frozen banana coated with dark chocolate and/or nut butter

➢ Dr. Tanya's Tip: A Pescetarian Diet

Some vegetarians also eat fish (I did during the fourteen years I was a vegetarian), which adds a great dimension to the diet. If you and your family eat fish twice a week, you likely won't have to worry about iron and B_{12} levels. While not all kids take easily to fish, if you cook, serve, and eat it early and often, your child will too.

Raising Children on a Vegan Diet

A vegan diet, one that excludes not only meat but also all animal products (such as eggs and dairy), can be extremely healthy, but it is critical that you ensure that your child is getting adequate calories and nutrients for proper growth and development. Let's consider a few issues that a vegan family needs to keep in mind.

In my practice I often see vegan toddlers or young children who aren't eating quite enough of the proper foods to support growth. For example, beans and brown rice are a wonderful source of fiber and protein, but some young children may not eat big enough servings of these to get sufficient calories and nutrients.

A young child needs many vegan fat sources for brain development and to sustain growth. It's a good idea to cook with plant-based oils such as olive and canola, perhaps use a vegan "buttery" spread on grains, and include lots of avocado and/or guacamole in your family's diet. Nuts are another wonderful, and vital, part of a vegan diet. Add nut butters, nuts, and seeds to meals and snacks frequently; they are a healthy source of protein and are calorie-dense. One of my healthy vegan families serves their children nuts first thing every morning.

Some plant foods are technically considered "incomplete" proteins when compared to animal foods. An egg, for example, has all the nine essential amino acids the body cannot manufacture itself but needs to function properly. Plant-based proteins such as beans or nuts do *not* have a high level of all nine essential amino acids. Specific protein combinations (such as beans and rice together) used to be recommended at each meal, but now we know that the body can generally forge what it needs as long as a vegan consumes a *variety* of protein sources throughout the day (not necessarily at each meal together) *and* the calorie needs are met.

Children need calcium and vitamin D for bone and immune system health, as we have seen. Offer your child three servings a day of soy milk, almond milk, or rice milk fortified with both calcium and vitamin D. It's important to note that soy milk contains a good amount of protein (equivalent to dairy milk), while the other milk alternatives do *not* contain enough protein for a young child to grow. (See chapter 3, "Milk Matters," for more discussion of various milks.)

It may also be necessary to supplement vitamins B_{12} and D, along with calcium, iron, and zinc. (See Dr. Tanya's Tip on daily multivitamins on page 190.) If your family is vegan and you would like your child to be vegan as well, talk to your pediatrician and a registered dietitian to create a healthy meal plan, and involve those experts as you carefully monitor your child's growth and development.

Vegan Meal and Snack Ideas

As always, the Eleven Foundation Foods are well represented in the list below. Be sure to modify these suggested options for your child's age and cut foods into small pieces (as needed) to prevent choking.

- Whole-grain waffle with a thick coat of nut butter
- Bean, brown rice, and avocado burrito
- Falafel and hummus with pita chips
- Corn tortilla heated with mashed kidney, garbanzo, or black beans, drizzled with olive oil
- Sliced apple with a thick coat of nut butter
- Nut-based trail mix (preferably a homemade, healthy mix)
- Salad with beans, sunflower seeds, avocado, and an olive oil–based dressing
- Lentil soup with brown rice or whole-grain pita chips
- Vegetarian chili made with beans, side of cornbread
- Baked potato with black or other beans, an olive oil drizzle, broccoli, vegan "buttery" spread

- Whole-grain toast with nut butter or mashed avocado
- Whole-grain cereal with soy milk

Going with the Flow

While there are many vegan families with absolutely thriving kids, a vegan diet doesn't quite work as well in certain children. For whatever reason, some vegan kids (as well as many kids who eat all sorts of foods) have trouble gaining weight adequately. If that's the case with your child, please work with a registered dietitian who has a vegan specialty to increase calories and protein so that your child can gain weight and grow appropriately.

Be innovative in trying new foods and experimenting with new preparations. I believe that it's vital, absolutely necessary, and non-negotiable (any other adjectives I missed?) that you learn to cook well and creatively if you plan to raise a vegan (or vegetarian) family! The rice-and-bean (or cheese quesadilla) options quickly get tiresome and alone can't provide all the nutrition your child needs.

Birth to age five is a special time of growth and development for the brain as well as the body, and while some adults can get away with a nutritionally lacking diet, kids absolutely require a balanced diet for proper development. This can be achieved with a well-planned plant-based diet as long as you check in with your pediatrician regularly to make sure that your child is gaining weight, growing appropriately, and getting all the nutrients needed to thrive.

Remember This

- It's possible to raise a healthy vegetarian or vegan child as long as you educate yourself about proper nutrition and ensure that your child is getting enough of all the nutrients needed to grow and develop.
- A proper vegetarian diet for a child is more than quesadillas. Include beans, lentils, all forms of nuts and seeds, eggs, and dairy products.
- A proper vegan diet for a child should include soy products, beans, lentils, nuts, seeds, avocado, and other healthy fats.
- Buy calcium- and vitamin D–fortified alternative milks. Soy milk is a better source of protein than nut-based milk alternatives.
- Work with your pediatrician to closely monitor your child's growth and development, and add supplements such as vitamin B_{12}, vitamin D, zinc, iron, and calcium if appropriate.

11.

Organic, GMO, and OMG

Just Tell Me What to Buy at the Store!

There's often confusion about how to make the best choices when it comes to the buzzwords we hear being thrown around about food: organic versus conventional, growth hormone–fed versus hormone-free, GMO versus non-GMO, local, in-season, etc. Let's break down what these concepts mean, discussing the benefits (some controversial) and the questions that they commonly raise for parents, and I'll weigh in on how to make the best nutrition choices for you and your family.

Organic Foods

If a food is organic, is it automatically the best and healthiest choice? If you can't (or don't want to) go completely organic, how do you decide which foods to buy organic or which to buy conventional? It's important to note that it's *your* budget and *your* choice, so please buy healthy food no matter what, and choose organic according to your personal preference and philosophy.

There are three common reasons why people buy organic foods: to lower pesticide consumption (and use), to reduce consumption (and use) of growth hormones and antibiotics in food sources, and to eat food that's generally perceived as "healthier." Let's look at each in turn.

Lower Pesticide Consumption (and Use)

Organic foods have stricter pesticide guidelines than conventional foods, which means fewer pesticides on the table. That's got to be a good thing. I firmly believe that organic foods are (1) better for our bodies and (2) more sustainable and better for the soil and environment. Though pesticide use is most often associated with fruits and vegetables, pesticides also end up, indirectly, in meat. That's because when pesticides are used on two extremely common components in our food supply, corn and soy, not only do *we* consume those items, but so do animals; animals take in the pesticides by eating their feed, and we get a dose by eating *them*. If you think of organic meat, you can see that it's more expensive in part because of the organic feed provided to the animals.

Here is the scoop straight from the U.S. Environmental Protection Agency: "Organically grown food is food grown and processed using no synthetic fertilizers or pesticides. Pesticides derived from natural sources (e.g., biological pesticides) may also be used in producing organically grown food."[19]

Why is it important to decrease pesticide exposure in children? According to expert Charles Benbrook, interviewed by the Center for Science in the Public Interest, "Pound for pound, children are exposed to more pesticides than adults. And their developing bodies are more sensitive to the adverse effects of pesticides."[20]

That said, it's important to know that eating fruits and vegetables (of any type) is good nutrition for you and your children. Don't avoid

> ➢ Dr. Tanya's Tip: **Buying Local and in Season**
>
> **It's a good idea to buy domestic produce that's in season in your own locale (such as cherries in the summer, not in February). According to the Center for Science in the Public Interest, "Roughly 80% of the average American's pesticide risk now comes from imported produce."[21] Produce from abroad, such as peaches and nectarines from Chile and sweet bell peppers from Mexico, has consistently high ratings of pesticide residue. Another important reason to buy local!**

a fruit or vegetable simply because it's not organic. If you buy conventional produce, just make sure you wash it well—for that matter, you should also wash organic produce well—and minimize your consumption of the foods highest in pesticide residue (see below for specifics). Peeling conventionally grown fruit can also help: fruits with skins that you peel or remove (such as watermelons and bananas) generally retain less pesticide residue than fruits with skins that you eat (such as strawberries and grapes).

Reduce Consumption (and Use) of Growth Hormones and Antibiotics in Food Sources

For a meat or dairy product to be USDA Certified Organic, producers must adhere to strict guidelines regarding the use of antibiotics, hormones, and various medications given to the animals. Buying organic gives your family potentially less exposure to all of these. In the grocery store, this may be a matter of budget and personal preference. The nutrients in dairy products and meat are important, whether organic or not. Kids still need the protein and iron in meat (or beans and lentils if vegetarian), and the calcium and vitamin D in milk, no matter what kind you choose to buy.

There's still much that scientists don't know for sure, but let's review what *is* known about growth hormone and antibiotic use in meat and dairy cows, to help you make educated decisions at the grocery store.

Many parents ask me whether hormones given to animals affect children who eat products made from those animals. First, a few basics. Have you ever seen "hormone-free" on a pack of chicken? I see this on "natural" packs of chicken all the time but it is false advertising because *all* chicken sold in the United States is hormone-free by law.

Q&A: Solutions for Real Parent Questions

Health-Conscious Family Foods on a Budget

Q: I want to cook healthy food for my family, but we're on a tight budget. What can I do?

A: You can still cook and eat nutritiously while keeping your budget in mind. Here are our favorite tips for feeding families on a budget:

- Take advantage of frozen fruits and vegetables, which are often lower in price but not in flavor. We love throwing frozen berries or other fruit into a smoothie, along with some plain or vanilla yogurt. You can add frozen spinach to lasagna, frozen leeks to soup, frozen bell peppers to quesadillas, and frozen corn to cornbread, pizza, or soup.
- Buy bulk containers of yogurt and cottage cheese. You'll save money and reduce packaging.
- Buy on-sale produce, which is usually in season as well. You can often find bananas, oranges, and apples at great prices.
- Try Trader Joe's, which carries many great products, including organics, at reasonable prices. Even their processed foods tend to

Straight from the USDA: "Hormones are not allowed in raising hogs or poultry."[22]

They *are* allowed in beef and dairy, however, and there are thousands of Internet articles warning against hormone-caused cancer, early puberty, endocrine disruption, lower IQ, and more. I would caution readers to closely examine the source of any article and the qualifications of the writer. Obviously people do have concerns: according to the AAP clinical report titled "Organic Foods: Health and Environmental

have fewer ingredients and fake colors compared to conventional markets. Those foods that carry the TJ's brand usually don't contain any artificial colors or artificial preservatives. (You can read more about their guidelines regarding additives on their website.)

- Buy store-brand versions of items like pasta.
- Buy potatoes and beans, which are good for you but often cheap.
- Freeze extra whole-grain bread or bagels and defrost as needed, so bread products don't go bad.
- For protein, you can often find great buys on chicken thighs and tuna.
- A whole chicken is generally less expensive than chicken parts. When you roast a chicken, serve it first on its own; then use the leftovers in soups and casseroles.
- Buy frozen fish, which tends to cost less than fresh.
- Buy frozen chicken breasts or thighs, often available in "value-size" packages at a lower price.

Advantages and Disadvantages," "Hormone supplementation of farm animals, especially with GH [growth hormone], is one of the major reasons consumers state they prefer to buy organic foods."[23] However, it's important to know that bovine growth hormone is biologically inactive in humans.

BETH'S GROCERY GUIDE

Conventional or Organic Milk?

I changed some of my views on dairy after visiting a farm in Wisconsin. The farmer took me on a long and extensive tour of his dairy farm. His operation is conventional, but he uses no hormones, and the milk his cows produce goes to cheese production in Wisconsin. My family and I petted the cows—even the adorable babies! Though this farmer's milk is produced conventionally, I felt fully confident about letting my children consume it.

I recently read a popular blogger's article demanding that a nationwide coffee chain switch to all-organic milk. I feel that this kind of demand warrants a discussion and understanding of our food supply. Perhaps not all the consumers of the coffee chain want to pay extra for organic milk. Perhaps there's not enough organic milk available to meet such a huge demand.

Organics are a result of consumer demand. The more consumers there are who demand organic food, and are willing to pay for it, the more will be available. But there is still a huge population that buys conventional milk, whether because of price or other considerations (such as supporting local dairy farmers).

Organic or not, milk is one of the Eleven Foundation Foods. Milk and the products made from it (yogurt, cheese, and so on) are health-promoting and nutrient-rich, and they're generally liked by children. Choose according to your personal beliefs and budget.

Dr. Louise Greenspan, in her book *The New Puberty,* explains that hormones found in milk and meat probably do not play a role in triggering puberty. This isn't an argument against buying organic milk and meat, because she does go on to say, "The real offenders are chemicals in the environment that, once ingested, act like hormones." Such "hormone mimickers," technically known as endocrine-disrupting chemicals, bind to estrogen receptors in the human body and may contribute to early puberty. "Endocrine-disrupting chemicals include antibiotics (found in meats and dairy products), bisphenol A (BPA), tobacco, phthalates, flame retardants, pesticides, and polychlorinated biphenyl compounds (PCBs)."[24] It's best to avoid these chemicals whenever possible in your family's food supply and environment.

Now, let's discuss the use of antibiotics. Studies have shown that "repeated exposure to broad-spectrum antibiotics at ages 0 to 23 months is associated with early childhood obesity."[25] This study found an "association." More research needs to be done on the relationship between antibiotics and early childhood obesity. If your child has a serious infection, she may need treatment with antibiotics, but why expose a child to unnecessary (nontherapeutic) antibiotics through the food supply? In addition, the AAP states: "Evidence is clear that such nontherapeutic use promotes development of drug-resistant organisms in the animals and that these organisms then colonize the intestines of people living on farms where this practice occurs. Evidence is also ample that human disease caused by antibiotic-resistant organisms spread through the food chain."[26] Presumably, then, buying organic (or at least antibiotic-free) meat decreases the threat of drug-resistant organisms in children.

As for milk, there are strict rules regarding the use of antibiotics in dairy cows, and the FDA requires frequent testing of milk for drug residues.[27] In 2015 the FDA tested almost two thousand dairy farms for drug residues in milk and found that "more than 99 percent of the samples [were] free of drug residues of concern—underscoring the safety of the US milk supply."[28] Yes, conventional dairy cows are allowed to have antibiotics when needed, but there are strict rules: milk can be released into the food supply only after treated cows have been off antibiotics long enough that their milk is clear of antibiotic residues.

For milk labeled USDA Organic, "the organic cow cannot be given growth hormones or antibiotics, and its feed must be 100 percent organic. . . . If it gets sick and needs treatment with antibiotics or other drugs, organic standards require that it receive these treatments but then must be removed from organic production. In other words, product from treated animals can no longer be sold, labeled, or represented as organic."[29]

Neither is a 100 percent perfect system, because the government cannot inspect every ounce of milk, conventional or organic, in our food

BETH'S GROCERY GUIDE

Purchasing Produce

1. BUY IN SEASON. If you want an out-of-season fruit like berries in January, there are many high-quality frozen options available. Avoid imported fresh produce from faraway places. I remember as a child the excitement of summer fruits coming to the grocery stores: watermelon, peaches, nectarines, apricots, and cherries. Kids these days don't learn what's in season because they see many of the same fruits and other foods year round. Take the opportunity to teach your children about seasonal foods.

2. BUY LOCAL. Ideally, the food you eat should be grown in your time zone. Local produce isn't always available, depending on where you live, but make an effort to purchase at least *some* locally grown items.

3. CHOOSE ORGANIC IF YOUR BUDGET ALLOWS. Eating fruits and vegetables trumps eating organic, but if you're looking for *which* fruits and vegetables to spend your organic food budget on, pay attention to the Environmental Working Group's (EWG) yearly "Dirty Dozen" guide. It changes slightly from year to year, but basically recommends

supply. While the U.S. milk supply is very safe, some experts do have concerns about chronic low-dose exposure to antibiotic residues.

What's the bottom line? Choose antibiotic-free meat whenever possible. It's a good idea to decrease your family's exposure to antibiotics and thereby help slow the spread of antibiotic-resistant illness. In addition, antibiotics may contribute to obesity, as noted earlier. A problem in its own right, obesity is also a major factor in early puberty.

Consider the source of all your meat choices. Fast-food meat is generally low-quality (and likely has hormones, antibiotics, and other things your kids don't need), while the organic and/or grass-fed beef that you buy at the store is of higher quality. And let's not forget that a

---

buying organic for soft-skinned fruits and veggies that you don't peel, such as strawberries and other berries, grapes, celery, peaches, pears, apples, and cherries.

The EWG's 2015 "Dirty Dozen" fruits and veggies—that is, those with the *most* pesticides—are apples, peaches, nectarines, strawberries, grapes, celery, spinach, sweet bell peppers, cucumbers, cherry tomatoes, sugar snap peas (imported), and potatoes. Each of these foods, when conventionally grown, tested positive for a number of different pesticide residues and showed higher concentrations of pesticides than other produce items. Most guides agree that it's okay to buy conventional for items with inedible skins or leaves that you discard, such as bananas, pineapples, and onions.

The EWG's 2015 "Clean Fifteen" fruits and veggies—those with the fewest pesticides when conventionally grown—are avocados, sweet corn, pineapples, cabbage, sweet peas (frozen), onions, asparagus, mangoes, papayas, kiwi, eggplant, grapefruit, cantaloupe, cauliflower, and sweet potatoes. You can find the latest EWG lists at ewg.org.

4. SHOP AT FARMERS' MARKETS. You'll hit the first two points, above, and be able to make your choice about number three.

BETH'S GROCERY GUIDE

Food Dyes

Food dyes are added to many processed foods. As we saw in chapter 9, they are "named" (on ingredient lists) with a color and a number, such as Red 40 or Yellow 5. It's a good idea to reduce chemical food dyes whenever possible. Controversy abounds over whether these dyes have negative health effects. Many of the dyes we use in the United States are banned in other countries. Chances are, foods with fake colors are also highly processed and have a long ingredient list. There are plenty of alternatives available that use natural methods of coloring, such as beet juice, turmeric, and other plant derivatives. These are healthier, more natural options.

Common culprits for food dyes include bright sugar cereal, fruit gummies and other fruit snacks, granola bars with candy pieces, oatmeal with candy pieces, and yogurt with cookie or candy toppings.

Food dyes also hook children on unnatural items that you can't replicate at home. I had a six-month unsuccessful mission of trying to replicate the taste and bright orange color of a popular brand of macaroni and cheese. My daughter always asks for the "more orange" brand, preferring it to my own "less orange" (but very tasty) recipe. She likes to order the "more orange" brand at restaurants. I try not to worry too much about that since she eats it infrequently; it's not a home "staple food."

Consumers are complaining about food dyes and major corporations are listening! General Mills announced in 2015 that they're removing artificial flavors, and colors from artificial sources, from all General Mills cereals. That's great news! Other companies are following their lead. The nationwide chain Panera Bread, for example, committed to removing a long list of additives/preservatives from their products. Chains such as Chipotle are proving that restaurants can be successful and responsible at the same time by sourcing local and non-GMO ingredients and limiting antibiotic and synthetic hormone use in their food.

plant-based diet has many health benefits, so think about cutting back on the quantity of meat you and your family eat, and instead go for occasional high-quality meat.

Eat Food That's Generally Perceived as "Healthier"

This rationale is controversial, because "organic" does not automatically equal "nutritious." Studies have shown mixed results: some have found no difference between nutrients (such as vitamin or mineral content) in organic and conventional food, while other studies have found small differences.

When it comes to organic *processed* foods such as cereal bars and cookies, "organic" may be screaming from the rafters—but that doesn't mean they're a healthy choice. There are plenty of thirty-ingredient cereal bars that are organic, but are still ultra-processed, low-nutrient foods. Many organic foods are indeed healthier—perhaps they don't have fake colors, are made from organic whole grains, and are minimally processed. But you can also find these characteristics in conventionally grown food. Reading labels and choosing wisely is key.

Is organic pasta a better nutritional choice than regular pasta? My

Family Feeding

Take your kids to your local farmers' market! It's a wonderful opportunity for them to learn how seasonal produce changes. Market vendors often give yummy free samples, and your child might be tempted to try something new. Our local farmers' market sells not only produce, but also free-range eggs, grass-fed meat, delicious balsamic vinegar glazes, dried fruits, nuts, and more. You'll support your local growers and enjoy fresh seasonal produce.

opinion is that there's probably little *nutritional* difference between the two. But often people purchase organic pasta for other reasons (such as environmental impact or personal philosophy).

When it comes to health and nutrition, the Eleven Foundation Foods and other one-ingredient foods are best. When it comes to nutrients, broccoli is broccoli.

Best Use of Your Organic Dollar?

Besides the three topics previously discussed (environmental concerns, growth hormones / antibiotics, and nutrition), you may have other

BETH'S GROCERY GUIDE

Navigating the Grocery Store

Here's a quick, aisle-by-aisle guide to making the best choices at the supermarket:

- CEREAL AISLE. Buy only products with at least 3 grams of fiber per serving, and no fake colors.
- BREAD/TORTILLA AISLE. Avoid bread with added "wheat gluten" and tortillas with fifteen to twenty ingredients. I love uncooked tortillas (sold in the refrigerated section) that you heat at home for thirty seconds per side. Remember: short ingredient lists and fiber are your friends.
- FROZEN FOOD AISLE. Pile on the frozen produce!
- JUICE AISLE. Skip the juice aisle altogether; don't go there!
- YOGURT AISLE. Buy no fake colors, no toppings. Yogurt with fruit on the side is fine. Greek yogurt is a good choice. Products with probiotics or live cultures are healthy for all.

beliefs that guide your choices at the grocery store. Most of us don't have an unlimited food budget, so choices and compromises are needed.

For Beth and me, the most compelling reasons to buy organic are (1) to avoid pesticides and care for the environment, and (2) to avoid hormones/antibiotics. The actual nutrient content of the organic versus conventionally grown food is less important to us.

Base *your* choices on your budget and your personal philosophy. Consider buying organic for the "Dirty Dozen" fruits and vegetables (see pages 206–07) and purchasing antibiotic-free meat. But the most important take-home message in this book is to feed your children the healthy, nutrient-rich Eleven Foundation Foods first.

- MILK AISLE. I prefer organic milk when possible; otherwise, I recommend that you buy local over national brands. I believe that chocolate milk is okay.
- CRACKER/CHIP/PRETZEL/POPCORN AISLE. Snacks with at least 3 grams of fiber per serving are ideal. You're almost certainly dealing with low-nutrient filler foods if items have zero or one gram of fiber. I love popcorn for older children (without added butter).
- CANNED FOOD AISLE. Go for canned beans and tomatoes—good value for good nutrition.

The sheer number of products at the grocery store is overwhelming. Next time you shop, take a look at the yogurt section to see what I mean! Even at a health-food store you can pile unhealthy foods into your cart. The most important grocery store message is: short ingredient lists.

The GMO Question

GMO stands for "genetically modified organisms." Scientists use genetic modification to introduce new traits or characteristics to an organism, often to address specific pest concerns or enhance crop yield. The most common GMO foods in the United States are corn and soy. Presently, GMO wheat is not allowed in our food supply. If you see "Made with non-GMO wheat" on a food label, that's a little misleading, because *none* of our wheat is GMO.

Generally speaking, though, it's not easy to avoid GMO products. Under current food-labeling regulations, GMO foods don't have to be labeled as such, though there's proposed legislation in several states to make labeling mandatory.

Scientists have yet to determine whether GMOs pose a health risk. However, there are still good reasons to avoid GMOs, perhaps most important the fact that there have been few safety studies on genetically modified foods, so we don't really know much about their effects.

Buying non-GMO products is a personal decision based on your own philosophy, preference, and food budget, as well as on information available to you. If you eat processed foods, it will be more difficult for you to avoid all sources of GMO. If you want to avoid or minimize GMOs, choose organic products (which aren't allowed to contain GMOs), choose products with various non-GMO certifications (such as Non-GMO Project Verified), and avoid processed foods with long ingredient lists.

If your head is still spinning, try not to stress about what your family ate last night, or last month; just make a pact that starting now you will focus more on nutrient-rich foods for your entire family. Choose wisely when it comes to organics, buy in-season fresh produce, take advantage of frozen produce for out-of-season fruits and veggies, think about reducing animal foods that use antibiotics, and avoid fake colors in your food to benefit your family, the environment, and hopefully generations to come.

Remember This

- Consider buying organic produce when possible, especially fruit with skins that you eat.
- Wash all produce well, but especially conventional produce.
- When you buy conventional produce, choose those with skins that you peel and the EWG's "Clean Fifteen." Minimize your purchase of foods highest in pesticide residue, such as the EWG's "Dirty Dozen."
- Choose organic, or at least antibiotic-free, meat and dairy, whenever possible.
- If you want to avoid or minimize GMOs, choose organic products or products with various non-GMO certifications.
- Always look for short ingredient lists and avoid foods with fake colors.
- There is little nutritional difference between many organic and conventional foods so buy nutrient-rich, healthy food first. Buy organic based on your budget and personal philosophy.

12.

Weighty Issues

The Underweight or Overweight Child

One thing all parents worry about at one time or another is their child's weight. Out of thousands of topics parents worry about, even weight worries can start early. You may start worrying about your child's weight before she can even sit up: the other babies in Mommy and Me are wearing nine-month clothes, and you're already browsing the toddler section for clothes that fit your little one; or the other toddlers look roly-poly and yours looks like skin and bones!

Even if your one-year-old looks like a future linebacker, it's not a good idea to put him on a diet. I promise you that the more you mess with your child's diet—restricting portions, serving "diet" foods—the *more* likely he is to gain excess weight. Beth and I believe that if parents serve the right foods (including the Eleven Foundation Foods), maintain (and encourage in your child) a reasonably healthy lifestyle, and impart a reasonably healthy attitude toward food, their children will generally reach a "just-right" weight.

In this chapter, I'll discuss how to help your child achieve his just-right weight; then provide solutions if he needs a little help achieving a healthy weight. Hopefully, this will calm any lingering worries and assure you that the feeding choices you are making for your child are giving him the proper nutrition for growth.

Growth Charts

Beginning right after birth, your pediatrician will start plotting your child's height and weight on standardized growth charts. In my practice I rely on those charts too. They help us identify trends and potential problems as a child grows; we never use them to assess a child's weight in isolation.

As a parent, *you* shouldn't look at weight in isolation either. For example, your child may be at the 5th percentile for weight on the growth chart. She's eating well and trying a great variety of foods. She stays on the 5th percentile for weight for most of her well-child visits. Her height remains at the 15th percentile. She's not underweight; she's just smaller in weight compared to most kids of her age. When you compare her weight to her height (also on the smaller side), her weight is within a normal range, or just right.

Now let's look at a young child whose growth curve is at the 90th percentile. She's active, eats well, and loves fruits and vegetables, but her parents are worried because she's bigger than many of her friends. Yet she's consistently followed along the 90th percentile weight curve (and likewise been at a consistent, high percentile for height) for years. She isn't overweight; she's at her just-right weight. It would be inappropriate and harmful to put this child on a diet, even though her weight is at the 90th percentile.

After age two, pediatricians start calculating a child's Body Mass Index (BMI), which is a ratio of weight to height. The BMI percentile is helpful, as are weight and height stats, in looking at growth *trends*. With a child you can't look at just one point in time for weight or height; you need to look at her entire growth history.

Growth charts can help us figure out potential problems when a child deviates from his or her usual curve. Note, though, that there are certain periods when it's more common for percentiles or growth patterns to change. For example, between nine and twelve months, an infant often gains proportionally less weight than he has been, which may translate into dropping percentiles on the growth chart. The reason for this is that many nine- to twelve-month-olds are newly:

- On the go (constantly rolling, crawling, pulling to stand, cruising, and possibly walking), and thus burning more calories
- Less interested in sitting down to eat for long periods of time, in part because they're more easily distractible
- Transitioning to self-feeding, and thus wanting to finger-feed independently—a hit-and-miss proposition—instead of allowing parents to spoon-feed

These three characteristics are all completely normal and often contribute to reduced weight gain during this time. In a child with any of these characteristics, a sudden change in growth trend is something that needs to be followed closely but isn't cause for panic. The child may catch back up in a few months, or may just be finding her new appropriate just-right spot on the growth curve.

In many cases of suspected excessive weight gain—say, kids jumping percentile categories (10th, 25th, 50th, and so on) in a year or two—we are able to identify some major change that contributed to either excess calories (eating more than his usual), lower energy expenditure (moving less than his usual), or both. For example, a young child who has always participated in sports stopped the previous year (or is off-season now, or took the summer off), and he's gained weight since becoming less active. Growth charts are great sources of information in cases like these, because we can ask, "Did something specific change between ages seven and eight?"

Just-Right Weight: The Traffic Light Strategy for Healthier Eating

Beth has been successfully using what she calls a traffic light system for years. I recommend it to you for kids of all ages. It allows you (and, equally important, your children) to start thinking about food in three simple categories: Green Growers, Yellow Fillers, and Red Reducers. Green Growers are the best choices—they're foods given the green light because they help kids grow—and you and your kids should look to choose most options from this category. Yellow Fillers are fine in moderation, so aim to combine some with your Green Growers. Red Reducers, as the "stop" color suggests, are foods that should be eaten and served most sparingly, as treats.

Green Growers

Serve Green Growers frequently. These items are one-ingredient foods, foods with a healthy, short ingredient list, or made-from-scratch foods. Our Eleven Foundation Foods are great examples of Green Growers. All of the following are Green Growers:

- Plain oatmeal you flavor yourself
- Higher-fiber cereals (at least 3 grams of fiber per serving) without fake colors
- 100 percent whole-wheat bread or other whole-grain breads/tortillas
- Whole-grain crackers (at least 3 grams of fiber per serving)

- Chicken
- Other lean meats
- Fish
- Beans/lentils
- Eggs
- Milk or soy milk
- Cheese
- Yogurt with no fake color
- All fruits, including plain dried fruit
- All vegetables
- All nuts and seeds
- Nut butters and seed butters without added sugar
- Air-popped popcorn or popcorn made with a small amount of olive or canola oil
- Natural applesauce

Yellow Fillers

Yellow Fillers have more ingredients than Green Growers; and those that are grain-based aren't 100 percent whole-grain. Serve one to two Green Grower foods alongside these foods to make a healthier meal or snack. Here are some examples of Yellow Fillers:

- Store-bought macaroni and cheese
- Plain white pasta
- White bread

- Store-bought cheese pizza
- Commercially produced granola bars
- Frozen prebreaded chicken tenders
- Crackers with 1–2 grams of fiber per serving
- Organic fruit leather or gummies with natural ingredients and no fake color

Red Reducers

Red Reducer foods are once-in-a-while foods, not daily foods. They include items such as the following:

- Fried foods
- Gummies or fruit rolls and fruit strips with fake colors
- Soda
- Juice
- Ice cream with fake colors
- Sugary breakfast cereals
- Toaster pastries
- Prepackaged "kid" lunches
- Frozen mini-bagels with toppings
- Chips with fake colors
- Frozen yogurt with candy toppings
- Most food marketed to kids!

A good message for children is that *all* food is okay, though it's not equally good for you. The traffic light system is an easy way to remember

➢ Dr. Tanya's Tip: Top Ten Ways to Help Your Child Achieve a Healthy Weight

1. **Be active.**
2. **Choose snacks wisely.**
3. **Monitor media.**
4. **Don't force a kid to clean her plate.**
5. **Resist food rewards.**
6. **Model healthy eating habits.**
7. **Take baby steps (small positive changes).**
8. **Cut liquid calories.**
9. **Serve nutrient-rich foods.**
10. **Remember that home-cooked is best.**

to serve and eat foods in the most nutritious way possible. Serve and eat green-lighted foods most often. Combine Yellow Filler foods with Green Grower foods to create a healthier combination. Serve and eat red-lighted foods least often, and in small portions. This will help both you and your child enjoy mealtimes!

Just-Right Weight Tips by Age

For all ages and many situations, I find it helpful to remember nutritionist Ellyn Satter's "division of responsibility" in eating that we discussed in chapter 5. Again, the division of responsibility means:

The parent's job is to prepare and offer food at appropriate times.

The child's job is to decide whether to eat (or not), and how much to eat.

Whether your child is underweight, normal weight, or overweight, you'll be fighting a losing battle if you try to control the amount your child eats.

Now let's take a look at some tips that will help you ensure that your child maintains her just-right weight.

Birth Through Age Two

- Let your baby meet you halfway, such as eagerly leaning forward in the chair to receive the food.
- Pay close attention to your child's "stop-eating" signals—such as turning her head away from the spoon and pushing back in her high chair.
- Offer many fruits and vegetables at most meals and snacks.
- Do not offer your child any juice, soda, or lemonade.
- Do not put your child on a fat-free diet. Healthy fat is *good*.
- Let your infant or toddler be in charge of amounts eaten. It is a rare child who cannot self-regulate appropriate portions at this age. If you're offering balanced meals and snacks (no fast foods, juice, or excess sweets), your child's weight should not be a concern.

Ages Three Through Four (Toddlers and Preschoolers)

- Frequently offer water in a cup.
- Strictly limit juice.
- Offer nonfat or 1 percent milk after age two, limiting the total to 16 to 20 ounces daily.
- Schedule sit-down snacks rather than letting your child graze on demand.

- Start healthy snack behaviors, such as having your child put a few whole-grain crackers into a bowl (rather than eating directly from the package).
- Limit restaurant meals, pizza delivery, and fried foods.
- Cook at home and eat family meals.
- Use healthy fats such as those found in nuts, olive oil, and avocado—don't put your child on a fat-free diet.
- Offer many fruits and vegetables—no limits on these!
- Set screen-time limits (see chapter 7 for advice about screen time) and encourage daily outdoor activity.

Age Five and Beyond (Elementary-Schoolers)

- Frequently offer water.
- Strictly limit juice and other sweetened drinks.
- Think about your child's schedule and leave her time for meals at home; when away meals are necessary, pack healthy meals to take with you. This is especially important when afternoons and evenings become jam-packed with activities.
- Offer nonfat or 1 percent milk.
- Offer high-fiber snacks, especially fruits and vegetables.
- Keep encouraging healthy snack behaviors, such as putting a few whole-grain crackers into a bowl (rather than eating directly from the package).
- Continue screen-time limits and daily outdoor activities (or fun indoor games during bad weather).
- Have reasonable limits on fried foods and pizza.
- Limit restaurant meals.

> ➢ Dr. Tanya's Tip: Sports Drinks
>
> **Water is the best thing for your child to drink during exercise. There are only a few rare, specific situations where a young child might benefit from a sports drink, such as a hard practice in hot weather, over an hour in duration. If you want to offer something other than water, low-fat chocolate milk is a better postgame option than a sports drink in most situations.**

- Have family meals.
- Offer and use healthy fats such as those found in nuts, nut butters, olive oil, and avocado—don't put your child on a fat-free diet.
- Make an after-school snack nutrient-rich so that your child is fueled for afternoon activities and homework (and can make it to dinner without added snacks). Many kids start wanting (and needing) a substantial snack or mini-meal after school at this age.
- Stick to water for sports; it's all that's needed 90 percent of the time. Discourage sports drinks.

Treating Overweight / Excess Weight Gain

When I see a child in my office who is overweight for her height, the first thing I do is take a detailed nutrition and activity history. I look for glaring problems such as soda, fast food, juice, inactivity, or too much screen time. If the family is eating wisely, exercising, and doing everything else right, and the child's physical exam is otherwise normal, I'm not usually concerned by a few extra pounds. Some kids go through phases when they gain weight more quickly, but eventually they "grow into their body." Genetics also plays a role: if either parent struggled with weight from a very young age, the child may face those same struggles.

More often than not, there's room for improvement: parents can bring a child's weight gain under control simply by making better food choices, decreasing sugar intake and portion sizes, increasing exercise, limiting screen time, and making sure the child is getting appropriate sleep.

Birth Through Age Two

When very young children seem to be gaining too much weight, it's important to look at their total calorie consumption and the foods they're eating. Do the following as well:

Monitor liquid calories. Juice, soda, and other unhealthy beverage items can be culprits in excess weight gain at this very young age. Bottle-fed infants may simply be consuming too much liquid. Work closely with your pediatrician to determine the proper amount of liquid nutrition, and make sure you're choosing drinks wisely.

Offer sensible snacks. Look closely at how you're doing in the snack-food category, and get in the habit of having healthy snacks such as fruits and vegetables around or offering snack-size portions of leftovers from nutritious meals.

Stick with nutrient-rich foods. Remember that this early age is the most critical time to build a healthy foundation for your child. Try to make every meal or snack nutrient-rich (including protein, dairy, whole grains, fruits, and veggies), and avoid getting your child used to the taste of unhealthy foods and drinks.

Ages Three Through Four (Toddlers and Preschoolers)

This is one of the easiest age groups to deal with, because you don't need to modify a young child's behavior as you do with older kids and teens. The key is modifying your *own* behavior in terms of what you're buying, cooking, and serving to your young child. Here are some tips to help you do that:

Shop wisely. For preschoolers, just stop buying offending foods such as cookies and chips—make them disappear from your house. Your kids may ask or beg or scream for a few days, and then they'll move on to healthier choices.

Monitor liquid calories. Stop drinking juice and soda (parents and kids alike). Instead, model drinking water and milk (even adults need calcium and vitamin D), and offer only those healthy beverages to your children.

Focus on parenting. Any behavior changes here should be 100 percent parent-focused. You can talk about healthy choices and portions, but it's really about the environment, caregiver behavior, and the foods and beverages that are available to the child.

Place no limit on fruits and veggies. I don't like telling kids they can't eat more if they're still hungry. If your child wants more food, please give it to her. But offer healthy options. In my house there are no limits on fruits and veggies! If you really think your child has eaten plenty and isn't truly hungry, try distracting her with a different activity.

Age Five and Beyond (Elementary-Schoolers)

Older kids, off at school and sports for much of the day, provide a greater challenge to parents concerned about potential excess weight. In addition to the suggestions for the previous age group, we recommend the following:

Don't resort to dieting. If an older child in my practice is gaining too much weight, generally I do *not* put him on a diet as a first-line option. Instead, I see if we can make healthy changes in nutrition and exercise, and help the weight stabilize as we let the height catch up. The last thing you want to do is start a child on a path of dieting, suffering, and deprivation, which inevitably leads to rebound overeating and mistrust of the whole feeding experience. Structured calorie restriction in a young child is very rarely appropriate; count calories only as recommended by your pediatrician.

Just because your child is bigger than his friends doesn't mean he has a weight problem. Work closely with your pediatrician and a registered dietitian to determine if there's something to worry about, or if your child is just following his normal growth curve for weight and height. Most important, where change is indicated, change how the *whole family* eats, not just one child! Healthier eating benefits the entire family.

Get help. Work with your pediatrician and/or a dietitian to try to determine the cause of your child's weight gain. Did it begin at a specific time? What else was going on in their life? Did physical activity change dramatically? Are there new caregivers? Was there a drastic change in the home?

Make your home a safe zone. Out of sight, out of mind. Buy primarily one-ingredient, nutrient-rich foods and choose packaged foods with shorter ingredient lists and no fake colors.

Limit excess calories. Offer your child water or milk to drink. If she's a juiceaholic and you're willing to support her habit, dilute the juice by at least half, and limit it to once a day. Think about where other excess calories may be lurking. Common culprits are parties and sports events with sugary treats, well-meaning friends and relatives who offer juice or soda to the child, too many restaurant meals, and too many food rewards. Limit all of these.

Try out the traffic light system. Use the strategy of categorizing foods as Green Growers, Yellow Fillers, and Red Reducers, as discussed above.

Place no limit on fruit and veggies. Serve many fruits and vegetables, and allow your child free access to these.

Apply the same rules for all. If there are other siblings in the house, the same rules should apply for all the kids. *No* child needs junk food; even skinny children don't need the extra fat and calories.

Focus on parenting, but involve your child. At this age, the intervention should still be parent-focused, although it's sometimes helpful to involve the child in the education process as well. Speak with your pediatrician and a registered dietitian to learn about healthy choices. It's important to note that at this age it's still not your child's fault. Don't expect him to take responsibility and decrease his servings or portion sizes. You can involve your child in making healthy choices, but keep the intervention parent- and family-focused.

Educate. You can teach your child about good nutrition, eating a variety of colors of the rainbow, and "brain hunger" versus "body hunger" (more on that later in this chapter).

Provide a distraction. Some kids get into the habit of eating when they're bored. When my son was having trouble with this, we would go into the backyard and kick the ball or play tag to distract him from eating and also to get in extra exercise activity.

Face restaurant realities. It's fun to go out and we all need a break from cooking once in a while, but the fact is that restaurants aren't well suited to kids' natural inclinations. Here are a few common problems and solutions to keep in mind when you take your kids out to eat.

PROBLEM: Kids will fill up on bread or chips while waiting for "real" food.

SOLUTION: Ask for bread or chips to be served *with* the meal instead of *before*—or, better yet, order a side of veggies to come first instead.

PROBLEM: Portions tend to be big. I estimate that the kids' pasta meal at our local Italian restaurant comes with 3 cups of angel-hair pasta!

SOLUTION: Ask for a meal to be split between multiple kids, or for a portion to be packaged "to go" even prior to serving.

PROBLEM: Fresh fruit and veggies often aren't included with a kid's meal.

SOLUTION: Ask for a side order of fruits or veggies that everyone can enjoy.

PROBLEM: Kids are tempted to order apple juice, lemonade, or soda, and these are often included in the price of a kid's meal.

SOLUTION: Have a family rule that you do *not* order sugar-sweetened drinks like lemonade or juice—parents included!

Using Food as a Reward

One of Beth's adult patients has struggled with his weight for many years. He vividly remembers food rewards—the smell, the anticipation, and all the feelings tied up with food. He struggles now with finding ways to deal with his emotions without turning to food.

Do your child a huge favor and come up with nonfood rewards as early as you can! As physician and obesity expert Yoni Freedhoff says: "It's a world where kids can't step on a blade of grass without being rewarded with a treat."[30] If food rewards were truly infrequent, reserved for special celebrations, there would be no problem with them; the issue is frequency. As your child gets older, you'll find that treats are fairly constant: after sports practices and games, at birthday parties, and as rewards for positive behaviors. During Beth's younger daughter's recent T-ball season, snacks that parents brought included donuts, cookies, sugar-sweetened juices, and sports drinks. All these extras add up to way too much sugar and excess calories. It would have been just as easy for those parents to bring cut-up fruit and pretzels instead of cookies, or 100 percent–juice popsicles rather than sugar-sweetened varieties.

By all means, celebrate special events, but the treat shouldn't always be food. When you want to reward your child, pick one of the ideas below (or create your own). The earlier you start, the better!

- Read a book together.
- Go to the bookstore or library and pick out a new book.
- Buy something from the dollar store.
- Go roller-skating.
- Take a bike ride.
- Play a game with Mom or Dad.
- Let your child choose an activity she wants to do for an hour.
- Give your child a free pass for an assigned chore.
- Take a walk together around the neighborhood.

Treating Underweight / Inadequate Weight Gain

Underweight kids may have poor weight gain, but that's not always a cause for concern. If a young child starts *losing* weight, however, that's typically a dangerous situation. A young child should not lose weight. Warning signs regarding underweight / inadequate weight gain include:

- Your child eats less or shows a marked decrease in appetite.
- Your child's growth slows down, as indicated by a significant percentile decrease in height and/or weight on her growth chart.
- Your young child *loses* any amount of weight.

Your pediatrician will monitor all of these signs and investigate whether your child is truly losing weight or not growing appropriately. Here are some specifics by age:

Infants

If your baby isn't gaining weight well, ask these questions:

- How is Mom's milk supply?
- How much liquid nutrition versus solid food is your infant consuming?
- Are there any medical concerns, such as swallowing issues, illness, or disease, that need to be treated?
- If your baby is taking formula, are you (and other caregivers) using the correct amount of water to mix the liquid?

Babies don't consume a huge volume of food, and sometimes—in a well-intentioned effort to give a child a very healthy diet—a parent might restrict fat too much. The advice for feeding an underweight baby is normally to cook with *more* healthy fat and to add calorie-dense or nutrient-dense items such as whole-milk yogurt, avocado, olive oil, and higher-fat meats and cheeses.

Toddlers

If your toddler isn't gaining weight well, ask these questions:

- Is your toddler drinking a low-calorie, low-protein milk substitute? Almond milk, coconut milk, and rice milk have fewer calories and protein, which can cause inadequate weight gain. (See chapter 3, "Milk Matters.")

BETH'S GROCERY GUIDE

The Danger of Highly Processed Foods for Self-Regulating Appetite

Our bodies are meant to self-regulate our appetite, food intake, and weight. But certain things get in the way—mostly habits, emotions, and highly appealing junk foods that mess with our natural regulatory system. Consider the following: compare how you would eat dry whole-wheat crackers versus cheese crackers stuffed with cheese filling.

As you've probably experienced, you'll eat only so much of a plain, dry cracker before stopping. But with a fatty, salty, slightly sugary cheese cracker, you'll keep going and going, ingesting hundreds more calories than your body really needs. To help with this tendency to overdo, choose foods with short ingredient lists and stay away from fake colors. Less-processed foods make it easier for children to regulate their appetite.

- Is your toddler getting a good balance of foods that contain carbohydrates, protein, and fat?
- Is your toddler filling up on too much milk, making him too full to want to eat solid foods?
- Are there any medical concerns, such as illness or an underlying medical condition, that need to be treated?
- Is there a feeding struggle or difficult dynamic between parent and child?

Preschoolers and Elementary-Schoolers

If your older child isn't gaining weight normally, ask these questions:

- How much milk (and what type of milk) is your child drinking?
- What does the rest of your child's diet look like?
- Is your child grazing or snacking all day on empty calories, preventing him from consuming proper, nutrient-rich meals?
- Is your child's diet too restrictive? Parents may feel like they're feeding their child the healthiest diet possible, but it may not contain enough protein, calories, or fat for adequate growth.
- Are you or your child avoiding certain food groups or nutrients; for example, are you eating gluten-free or dairy-free? If you need or want to eliminate a certain food group, it's important that you work with your pediatrician and/or a registered dietitian to ensure that your child is getting appropriate nutrients.
- Is there any underlying medical condition that needs to be treated?
- Is a busy schedule interfering with mealtimes?

- Is your child taking a medication that may decrease appetite? If so, this can often be managed quite well with the assistance of your pediatrician.

Brain Hunger vs. Body Hunger

Parents struggle when a child says she's still hungry after a meal or snack, especially when there's a weight concern. I don't like to withhold food from a hungry child—period. But thinking about how she feels in terms of "brain hunger" versus "body hunger" can help a child hold off for a bit.

Here are some options you can use to teach your child about brain hunger versus body hunger:

- EXPLAIN THAT THE BRAIN RUNS MORE SLOWLY THAN THE TUMMY. It's fine to tell a child that when people eat very quickly, their brain needs to catch up to their body. Older kids may benefit from waiting five to ten minutes, then having seconds if they're still hungry.

- OFFER FIVE MINUTES OF FUN. For a child who has trouble self-regulating and seems to be an empty bucket, try distraction for five to ten minutes with a fun after-meal activity. My oldest son would eat anything and everything and continue until we physically removed him from the table. Now that he's older, he's very capable of choosing healthy, appropriate portions on his own.

- RESPECT YOUR CHILD'S HUNGER AND FULLNESS SIGNALS. Young children have the ability to self-regulate their food intake. Encourage kids to determine when their tummy is full, and respect when they say they're either hungry or full.

- GIVE PROTEIN TO KEEP KIDS FEELING FULL. For "bottomless pit" kids, try offering protein-rich meals and snacks such as peanut butter with an apple, cheese with crackers, half a tuna sandwich with carrots, turkey slices with an orange.

- ALWAYS ALLOW EXTRA VEGGIES AND FRUITS. You may find that when you offer a still-hungry child veggies, he isn't really that hungry anymore! Worst case is he eats tons of veggies or fruits and gets tons of nutrition! I've never met anyone who gained weight because he ate too many fruits or vegetables.
- REASSURE YOUR CHILD THAT THERE WILL BE MORE. Beth's older daughter often waits too long to eat and doesn't realize how hungry she is. In that super-hungry state, she starts eating and announces that she wants more even before she's done with her first helping. Beth's response is, "I'm happy to make you more. Let's see how you feel when you're done with this." That's a much better response than, "Well, if you ate when you were supposed to, *blah, blah, blah.*" That kind of response only frustrates a young child.
- SEEK HELP. If you're concerned that your child constantly seems to be hungry, discuss your concerns with your pediatrician and/or dietitian.

Exercise

Kids need at least one full hour of exercise every day. Try to incorporate it into your family routine so that going outdoors and running around or just being active is a normal part of everyday life. You can certainly break the exercise up into smaller amounts a few times a day, such as a morning walk, an after-school soccer playdate, and an afternoon family dance competition. Just like good nutrition, healthy exercise habits start at a young age. *You* are your children's best role model, so let them see you exercising too!

Here are some family-friendly activities to get everyone moving:

Birth Through Age One

From day one you can place your newborn on a blanket on the floor and let her stretch; give her a few minutes of tummy time too, and watch her learn to lift her head and later push up and eventually begin to roll. Take her outside to explore. Let her crawl and later walk around on the soft grass. Get her used to being outdoors in the fresh air, but don't forget sun protection (UV clothing, hats, sunglasses, and sunscreen). Weather not cooperating? Chase her around the house acting silly. She will love it!

Ages Two Through Three

Toddlers thrive on unstructured play! Swinging, climbing, and playing in the sandbox are fun and healthy activities. Join in! They love playing with Mommy and Daddy, and you'll get some exercise too. Most toddlers are not yet developmentally ready for competitive activities, but they love to run and later kick or throw a ball. Keep in mind, if your child isn't interested in a specific activity, don't force it.

Ages Four Through Five

With increasing coordination, four- and five-year-olds can play catch and take part in other organized games such as soccer or T-ball. Individual activities such as karate, biking, and swimming are also great options. Remember that children this age still lack judgment, safety awareness, and coordination; thus they need to be closely supervised.

Safety Tip

Protective Gear: Make sure your children use protective gear such as helmets, and always watch your children when they're on playground equipment or near a pool or other water.

Through a combination of exercise, an active lifestyle, and good eating, your child should eventually reach the optimum weight for his body type. As we've seen in this chapter, when it comes to kids and weight, it's not the number on the scale that matters most, but the nutrition that your child is consuming day to day. Each sip and every bite makes a difference in terms of your child's overall health. Instead of focusing on what your child *shouldn't* be eating, focus on what he *does* need to eat to grow, to develop, and to form healthy habits for life. It's okay if your child doesn't fit perfectly on the growth chart, as long as he's getting proper nutrition. And if you find that your family needs assistance in making nutrient-rich changes, ask for help from your pediatrician and/or a registered dietitian. It often takes a village to raise a healthy child.

Remember This

- Base food decisions on the knowledge that what your child is eating and drinking is more important than your child's weight.
- Choose nutrient-rich foods with short ingredient lists and no fake colors, and try implementing the traffic light system with your family.
- Divide feeding jobs appropriately. The parent's job is to prepare and offer healthy food at appropriate times. The child's job is to decide whether to eat (or not), and how much to eat.
- Avoid using food as a reward.
- Build exercise activity into your family's daily routine.

13.

The Feeding Fix

Overhauling Bad Advice in Baby-Feeding Trends

Whether you're new to this parenting thing, or you're feeding your fourth child, you've probably encountered an overabundance of ideas, trends, and advice about the best way to feed your baby. Your friends might be throwing around phrases such as "baby-led feeding" and "only green food for the first year"—and you're just doing your best to get a nutritious dinner on the table every night!

Whether you're consulting books or the Internet, it can be hard to know which advice is best, and which should be avoided. That's part of the reason I wanted to write this book. Through my pediatric work, and in my relationship with the AAP, I've determined the best, safest, and most proven ways to feed your child. Let's take a look at a handful of feeding trends and explore the good parts . . . and the worrisome. Then I'll give you a way to take what's positive about each trend and use it in coordination with the advice I'm setting out in this book, so that you can rest assured you're feeding your child well.

Trend: Baby-Led Feeding

Made popular by such books as *Baby-Led Weaning*, by Gill Rapley and Tracey Murkett, this trend lets babies self-feed from the start, rather than parents initially spoon-feeding them purees. Instead of starting with traditional pureed foods, babies on this regimen start with finger foods, large pieces of foods, and even whole fruits or vegetables.

The Great

There is one goal that I share with the proponents of baby-led feeding: to encourage babies to eat healthy table food with the rest of the family as soon as possible.

The Worrisome

The premise of this trend is irresponsible and potentially dangerous, with little research to back up the advice. The above-mentioned book says that your baby "may suck at spaghetti, shovel rice or minced meat into her mouth, *gnaw at chicken bones,* try eating straight off the plate . . . or pick up peas one by one" (italics mine).[31] Gnaw at chicken bones? Raise your hand if you think it's safe for a six-month-old to gnaw on a chicken bone.

What worries me most is choking hazards! Here's a great example: "Offer your baby three or four different things to start with—maybe a piece of carrot, a broccoli floret, *and a large strip of meat*" (italics mine).[32] Babies are not small adults. They lack good judgment: they will put a button, magnet, toy, or *anything* nearby into their mouths. They cannot yet be trusted to fully feed themselves or determine what is or isn't a choking hazard.

Lastly, babies that are completely self-feeding will likely not get adequate calories or specific nutrients (such as iron) to support growth during this crucial time.

The Fix

As I explained earlier, parents *do* need to pay close attention to their baby's cues as she eats, and not just shovel in spoonful after spoonful of food. And it's important to advance beyond purees to thicker, lumpier items and then finger foods as soon as your baby can handle them. If you would like to try early self-feeding with your baby, the best, safest way is to put a few very tiny, soft bites near your baby and let her explore.

Pureeing itself, especially early on, is not wrong. Feel free to puree a little bit of whatever healthy food you're eating to provide your baby with nutrition until she's able to self-feed. It's important to control the self-feeding, however—to avoid choking hazards, as well as to make sure your child is getting adequate nutrition. As I explain to parents who follow baby-led feeding, your infant doesn't get nutrition simply by *licking* zucchini. And please, no gnawing on chicken bones or large strips of meat!

Trend: Vegetarian and Vegan Diets for Babies and Toddlers

I fully support eating a more plant-based diet, but as discussed in chapter 10, parents need to take special care when feeding children that type of diet. There are many varieties of vegetarian and vegan diets for kids, some responsible and some not. One popular, massive (672-page) book has a cult-like following; interestingly, it's a vegetarian book without overtly *saying* it's a vegetarian book.[33]

The Great

A good vegetarian or vegan feeding book emphasizes nutritious foods such as beans, whole grains, fruits and veggies, nuts, and seeds. It provides amazing meal and snack ideas for each family's specific needs. In addition, the plans are generally extremely supportive of breast-feeding.

One popular book in this category is Alicia Silverstone's *Kind Mama,* which encourages nutritious, "kind" foods from the start: "Babies don't come out of the womb only wanting to eat [cereal] and chicken fingers."[34] I agree!

Some books offer a grain-based porridge recipe for baby's first food, rather than packaged infant cereal; emphasize the rich, creamy, naturally lumpy consistency of home-prepared baby foods compared to jarred; and encourage parents to make their own baby food when possible. These are all great practices that I encourage parents to use with their children.

The Worrisome

The most worrisome part of this trend, and some others, is that the authors don't always have the credentials to be making the health claims that they do. Be very wary of unfounded statements and promises. One book with an anti–Western medicine viewpoint discourages fever reducers and other medications pediatricians use for certain childhood illnesses. I strongly recommend discussing any health-based decisions such as medical treatment with your pediatrician. Another book includes unconventional advice: "Your blender and food processor give off a lot of EMFs (electro-magnetic fields), so don't stand very close to it."[35] I haven't read anything that makes me concerned about standing in front of my blender.

Beware of unfounded statements such as, "Bananas in particular, though rich in vitamins, are a naughty food for baby and should be had in moderation."[36] Fruit is a wonderful and healthy food you should serve frequently. Another example is: "Jarred baby foods are made at such high heat that any vitamins once in that all-natural, organic container of butternut squash have been nearly obliterated (and then added back in artificially)."[37] This is a pretty broad statement with little factual backup.

Two especially dangerous things to watch out for are recommendations for homemade formula and recipes that call for raw milk. Check with your pediatrician before starting any homemade formula or using raw milk, to ensure that the foods you're considering contain the right balance of nutrients and are safe for your baby to consume. Raw milk may contain bacteria or other organisms, potentially deadly to young babies, that have not been killed by the heat of pasteurization.

Some plans may warn against feeding your baby (or yourself) foods made from dairy, fish, eggs, meats, and processed ingredients. However, these foods *can* be extremely healthy, especially dairy foods such as yogurt and milk. Yes, you can be a healthy vegan or vegetarian family, but you can also be a healthy family who eats chicken, fish, and other lean meats.

The Fix

Enjoy the many awesome baby-food recipes in vegetarian and vegan books, but as soon as your baby can advance beyond purees, move beyond them. Many books share hundreds of baby-food recipes, but remember that you need only a few. In the time it would take your baby to try all of those recipes just once, he would be out of the pureed stage and starting to transition to what the rest of the family is eating. Choose your favorite few recipes and roll with them. And if you don't want to go *totally* vegetarian, you can always use vegetarian baby-food recipes and add chicken, fish, turkey, and/or red meat as desired.

A few of these books make pseudoscientific claims presented as facts. If using these books, I recommend doing some research on any such claims, or discussing them with your pediatrician. You can also use those books alongside this book, to ensure proper nutrition and safety practices. I wouldn't hang my hat on any promises to cure disease. No need to add a pinch of kelp or desiccated liver, as one book recommends, to your baby's food! After age one, switch your mental focus and energy to making *family* meals, not making special food for the kids. Work very closely with your pediatrician to ensure that your child is growing and progressing well.

Trend: Gluten-Free Kids

The G-word has many moms and dads turning to a restricted-grain diet, but now some parents are also restricting gluten in their baby's and child's food.

The Great

Some of the gluten-free websites for feeding babies and children encourage other whole foods, such as potatoes, sweet potatoes, brown rice, and quinoa. These resources also advise limiting "white foods" such as highly processed gluten-containing bars and crackers with no fiber and long ingredient lists. I agree with both pieces of advice.

The Worrisome

Whole grains are an important part of an infant's and young child's diet, so removing all gluten-containing products leaves a big hole. Recent research shows that delaying introduction of gluten to infants does *not* decrease their chance of developing celiac disease later in life.[38] There is no reason to eliminate gluten unless your child has a documented allergy or celiac disease and you have discussed the plan with your pediatrician. (For more information on gluten allergies and celiac disease, see chapter 8.) Overall, babies and children should follow the least restrictive healthy diet possible.

The Fix

Limit "white foods" such as highly processed gluten-containing bars and crackers with no fiber and long ingredient lists. But don't eliminate gluten altogether. Instead, offer healthy whole grains such as whole wheat, oats, barley, rice, and more. Remember: whole grains make up one of our important Eleven Foundation Foods! There's no reason to eliminate gluten from your baby's diet unless he has celiac disease or some other documented medical issue.

Trend: Breast-feeding Exclusively Beyond Six Months Without Starting Solid Foods

Some moms so strongly believe that breast milk is the absolute best that they delay introduction of solid foods until their baby is nine to twelve months old.

The Great

Breast-feeding provides your baby with all the nutrition, antibodies, and other benefits of breast milk.

The Worrisome

Delaying introduction of solid foods can mean that your infant misses the window of learning how to eat solids, and the nutrition that comes with those varied foods. Around six months of age, infants need extra iron and zinc beyond what's provided in breast milk. Iron and zinc are very important for a child's developing brain, as I've noted before. In addition, delaying introduction of solids beyond six months may increase your child's risk for food allergies (see chapter 8). Finally, it's important to introduce your baby's palate to the distinct tastes and textures that only solid foods offer.

Although many infants will continue to prefer liquids to solids and may not show interest in eating food, they may have inadequate nutrient intake and weight gain on their liquid diet. Some argue that in many countries babies get little food besides breast milk until a much later age. While this is true, it is often out of necessity, not when food is in abundance.

The Fix

Continue to breast-feed as long as you wish; however, also gradually introduce solid foods, especially the Eleven Foundation Foods, starting around six months of age, using chapter 4 as a guide. If your baby is breast-feeding multiple times at night after six to nine months of age, watch out for liquid calories displacing calories from solid foods (as well as Mom's lack of sleep!).

Trend: Only Green Food for the First Year

This feeding trend advises only green vegetables until babies reach age one. It's common in some vegan and vegetarian communities.

The Great

Eating only green foods certainly exposes babies to healthy green veggies early and frequently.

The Worrisome

Although green vegetables do contain some iron, infants don't eat large enough quantities to get the amount of iron they need for proper growth and development. Protein and other important nutrients may also be missing from the diet of an infant who is eating only green vegetables. Lastly, the baby will not get used to eating other important foods during the critical window of introduction between six and twelve months of age.

The Fix

Feed plenty of green vegetables, but also offer the other Eleven Foundation Foods for iron, protein, fiber, B vitamins, minerals, and healthy fats. Include fruits too! By offering a variety of healthy flavors and textures, you're setting your child up to eat nutritious food for the rest of his life.

Trend: Sneaking Vegetables and Fruits into Other Foods

Craving black beans in your brownies, or cauliflower in your macaroni and cheese? Books such as *The Sneaky Chef* by Missy Chase Lapine and *Deceptively Delicious* by Jessica Seinfeld offer recipes, tips, and tricks to "sneak" nutritious ingredients into kid-friendly foods.[39]

The Great

"Sneaky" cookbooks have many nutritious recipes, they emphasize home cooking, and they provide make-ahead ideas for preparing a variety of pureed ingredients.

The Worrisome

The whole premise behind "sneaking" is that kids don't eat health-consciously enough and need an intervention. If a parent is worried that a child isn't eating enough fruits and veggies and feels that she needs to get these foods into him another way, her mind-set violates the "division of responsibility" in feeding. Now you, not the child, are trying to take charge of how much of a certain food he eats.

Older kids, more aware than babies, may get mad if a parent tries to sneak what they see as questionable food into other food, and become distrustful of *everything* that's served. Deception and sneakiness aren't high on my list of must-do parenting skills.

As important as it is for children to be eating healthy, nutritious food, it's also important for them to be exposed to various foods in their natural, recognizable state, so that as those children get older, they know they enjoy eating those foods and will *choose* to eat them. When a food is consistently hidden in something else, children won't know they like it, so down the road the strategy may cause some picky eaters.

The Fix

If you want to add pureed fruits or veggies to recipes, do it for the right reasons. Do it because it adds a great color or taste or different dimension to a recipe, along with the extra nutrition it provides. Whether or not you're adding purees, make sure you're also offering plenty of regular fruits and veggies in their natural form—but without pressuring your child to eat them. This way, your child is introduced to a food's natural taste and texture, and will grow accustomed to it and enjoy it.

That said, there's nothing wrong with bumping up certain recipes with extra fruits or veggies. Some easy ideas include:

- Adding pureed carrots, cauliflower, or butternut squash to mac and cheese
- Adding pureed bananas or applesauce to bread or muffins
- Adding greens to smoothies
- Adding shredded or minced carrots, zucchini, and/or other veggies to marinara sauce, meatballs, meatloaf, or pizza

Try recipes that include healthy ingredients without being deceptive, such as:

- Oatmeal-raisin cookies

- Banana bread or muffins
- Homemade tomato, pasta, or pizza sauce
- Fruit smoothies
- Recipes that are cooked with onions, garlic, or mirepoix (a combination of onions/celery/carrots)
- Blueberry muffins or pancakes

Trend: Food in Pouches

Many baby-food products are now sold in pouches rather than jars. A quick glance around the local mall or playground will show countless babies and toddlers slurping their lunches from a pouch.

The Great

Pouches are indeed convenient for parents on the go, and they're less messy for infants and toddlers to quickly suck down. Many are made by organic baby-food companies and have fruit and veggie ingredients. My older kids like them too!

The Worrisome

The food in pouches doesn't always provide the best nutrition for your infant or toddler, nor does it encourage the best eating behaviors. It can cause overeating, because kids practically inhale their food. Furthermore, slurping fruits and veggies doesn't get infants or older children used to eating actual, real fruits and veggies.

Even though many pouches tout organic fruits and veggies, a closer look often reveals a higher sugar content than in actual produce, and pediatric dentists worry that the sticky consistency may increase tooth decay. If you do choose to buy some pouches, make sure you read the ingredients carefully; often the fruit or vegetable listed on the front is only one of the dozen ingredients listed on the back, which means a miniscule amount of the fruit or veggie is actually in the pouch. Some pouch products include grains—one claims to "evoke the flavor of warm oatmeal." Instead of a pouch for breakfast, I suggest just making oatmeal. It doesn't take much longer, and the benefits are greater.

Grain pouch mushes often have many ingredients that just aren't necessary—especially for older babies and toddlers, who should be having solids, not mush! Pouch companies use "health halo" marketing strategies, such as including trendy grains like quinoa, Kamut, chia seeds, and more—but the foods are still mush!

The Fix

Use a spoon! Squirt a bite of the pouch contents into your spoon and feed it as you would regular baby food. If I'm out with only a pouch, I'll order a side of avocado, fork-mash it, add a little of the pouch puree, and spoon-feed the mix to my eight-month-old. Alternatively, purge the pouches completely and simply carry mashed, and later chopped, fresh fruits and veggies in a small reusable container. That's truly the best way to ensure that your child will grow up to enjoy eating actual fruits and vegetables. If you do buy pouches, choose those with fewer than five ingredients. Remember that just because it comes in a BPA-free pouch and is organic, that doesn't guarantee it's a healthy choice.

Trend: Mesh Nets for Baby Feeding

These baby feeders are mesh nets attached to a handle, to hold fresh solid foods such as apple slices or melon cubes. The food pieces go into the mesh pouch, it snaps shut, and the baby can suck on the mesh net with the food trapped inside.

The Great

Mesh nets decrease choking hazards, as the net allows only very tiny pieces of food (along with the natural juices and flavor) to come through. They can help train your infant's palate to enjoy the taste of healthy foods such as fruits and veggies. Nets can also be used to help teething infants gnaw on a cube of cold melon or other cold food.

The Worrisome

Simply mashing or pureeing food is easier for feeding your baby an actual meal, and she'll get more nutrition without working as hard. In addition, some parents report that the net is hard to clean.

The Fix

Use a net to allow your baby to explore the taste and flavor of various fruits and veggies without having to worry about a chunk breaking off and potentially becoming a choking hazard. When it's time for a meal, puree or mash and actually feed your infant the food; don't make her suck it through a net. Nets are fine for occupying your child and soothing teething discomfort, but they're not an effective way to deliver needed calories.

Trend: Prechewing Your Baby's Food

Technically called "premastication," this trend recommends that parents prechew all food and gently place it in their baby's mouth.

The Great

If you're stranded in the wilderness (or on a trip) with no other way to safely feed your baby solid food, prechewing does make sense as a way to mash food into a consistency your infant can eat. Many cultures without our modern conveniences of high-powered blenders and food processors don't have the luxury of pureeing food. They prechew food out of necessity, not because it's trendy.

The Worrisome

Prechewing your baby's food can transfer harmful adult bacteria from your mouth to your infant's mouth, increasing her chance of later dental cavities. In addition, children need to develop the skills of chewing, which they (obviously) develop by chewing gradually lumpier consistencies. Oh, and there's the gross factor.

The Fix

Instead of putting food in your mouth to prepare it for your child, simply put it in one of the many modern conveniences we now have, such as a blender or a baby-food grinder, or fork-mash it, then feed it to your baby.

Parents today have more advice than they'll ever need at their fingertips. Use this book as you navigate other feeding books and trends to determine the healthiest and safest way for you to feed your baby. The goal is to introduce and feed your baby a variety of nutrient-rich options that will promote not only proper growth and development now, but also good health and appropriate eating behaviors for life.

Remember This

- There are many trendy feeding plans on the market today. Do your research to determine which ones are backed by credible sources.
- Safety first! Make sure your feeding plans avoid foods that might be a choking hazard.
- If you choose one of these feeding plans, be sure to also include foods from the Eleven Foundation Foods to ensure a well-rounded, healthy diet.

14.

The Picky Eater

Preventing and Taming Five Common Picky-Eating Problems

Are you a POP—Parent of the Picky? Picky eating is a very common concern for parents, and a very common mind-set in kids! Luckily, there are many solutions to prevent or tame pickiness in young eaters. Join my POP support group, where we learn to alter our own behavior rather than catering to our Little Picky Person! If not handled properly, picky eaters can rule the roost.

Most POPs are surprised to hear that taming a picky eater, or preventing pickiness from ever taking root, isn't hard; it just takes patience and perseverance. But I promise that your efforts will pay off. To prevent and treat a picky eater, the most powerful tool at your disposal is this: serve your child what the rest of the family is eating.

Normal or Problem Pickiness?

Just as you may prefer your coffee at a certain temperature, your eggs soft but not runny, or your steak a certain degree of doneness, your child also has specific preferences. It's part of what makes your child so unique and wonderful!

There are some food quirks or preferences that it's fine to honor—as long as they don't cause you extra trouble or start ruling the household. For example, as a small child a cousin of mine liked marinara sauce very smooth, without chunks. My aunt would make sauce, then quickly puree some for her daughter, leaving chunks in what the rest of the family ate. No problem there. Beth often makes a slow-cooker Italian chicken that ends up with a sauce; her kids don't love "saucy" chicken, so either she or they simply blot away any sauce with a napkin. Perhaps your daughter wants her sandwich cut into triangles or the crusts cut off, or your son doesn't want any food touching other foods on his plate. To me these variations are acceptable, because it's the same food and doesn't cause much extra work. (You may feel differently.) On the other hand, you absolutely should not have to make multiple meals to satisfy your family's demands.

Standard picky preferences aren't always a problem that needs to be fixed. However, the parent's response can determine the road ahead—do you prepare one meal and let your child manage her preferences within that meal, or do you become a slave to catering to her preferences? You know that her preferences are getting out of hand when:

- The pickiness causes you extra work that's now a burden (for example, instead of a few seconds to cut a sandwich into triangles, you make something totally different).
- You have anxiety about taking the child to a situation in which unfamiliar food will be served.
- Your child becomes ultra-demanding and refuses to eat what the rest of the family is having.

Pickiness is a continuum, like most other child behaviors. Parents of toddlers often tell me, "Oh, he doesn't like that food," but then I learn that they offered it only a couple times before giving up. Parents need to

➢ Dr. Tanya's Tip:
Picky Eater vs. Problem Feeder

Unlike standard picky eaters, serious problem feeders aren't following normal child development. Here is a chart to help you identify whether your picky child has a feeding issue that needs to be evaluated by your pediatrician and possibly a feeding specialist.

Picky Eater	Problem Feeder
May be picky but ultimately eats enough calories a day to maintain healthy weight and growth	Has difficulty eating enough food and calories to grow and gain weight properly; may have other medical or behavioral issues
Eats fewer than thirty foods	Eats fewer than ten to twenty foods
May stop eating a favorite food, but will go back to eating it after about two weeks	Refuses to eat even favorite foods
Eats a limited variety, but will eat at least one food from each food group and each texture category (soft, crunchy, chewy, etc.)	Refuses entire categories of foods or foods with certain textures altogether
Will accept new foods on the plate and will at least touch or taste them	Regularly cries, screams, or throws tantrums when new foods are placed on the plate
Will eat new food (at least one bite) after a dozen exposures	Doesn't learn to eat any new foods even after twelve exposures, or won't try them at all

understand that it takes at least a dozen times for a child to accept a new food. You have to take the time to keep introducing it daily or weekly, and let your child see *you* eating it as well. If you don't eat the broccoli, he is much less likely to eat the broccoli.

An interesting study found that a powerful predictor of a child's vegetable intake was . . . wait for it . . . the parents' vegetable intake! Besides what the authors of that study called "parental modeling," availability and accessibility were also shown to be important. In other words, kids did better when produce was just plain available for eating, as well as easy for them to eat (already washed, peeled, and cut).[40] Taste is also a powerful ally at your disposal. Kids aren't motivated to eat *virtuous* food; they enjoy food that tastes good to them, so offer them good-tasting food whenever possible.

Some kids don't mind trying new things, but some are truly anxious and worried about new foods. Do not force your anxious child to swallow something they do not like. It creates a feeding battle, and your child has already made up his mind to hate that food. It is fine to encourage, and even to hold a fun taste test, but if your child is very worried about trying a new food, you will be better off not forcing. Beth's cousin was forced to eat carrots he hated in elementary school, and he will still never touch a carrot—at age fifty!

Kids also go through phases, and taste buds and preferences change. In my house we talk a lot about how taste buds change as kids get older; I'll bring this up when I introduce a food item that they previously didn't like. My middle son might say, "Mom, I think my taste buds changed because I don't dislike _____ (fill in the blank) food anymore." Or, if I'm lucky, he says, "I now like _____ (fill in the blank) food."

Below, we'll take a look at the five most common picky-eating problems, and I'll give you strategies for how to prevent and cure them. Over and above these strategies, my advice to parents is this: be patient. As I've said before, it can take a child at least a dozen times to accept a new food; and six to twelve months of intervention are often needed before a dedicated picky eater will begin to accept a wider variety of food.

1. Picky Produce Eaters

Many kids eat just one or two fruits or veggies and refuse to try any others. If your kid is one of them, don't suggest eating less of the fruit or veggie she likes. Instead, persistently serve other fruits and/or veggies at the same time. Worry less about her actual consumption; focus more on offering produce and eating it yourself. Just keep offering in a positive way (don't force!), keep modeling, and try to offer different fruits at many times of the day (without pressuring the child).

The theme for fruits and vegetables should be, "All fruits, all vegetables, all forms."

Some fun ideas to encourage your child to eat fruits and veggies include:

- Make smoothies and let your child help add the ingredients to the blender. True story—Beth made smoothies for at least four years before her oldest daughter would actually drink them. She finally started drinking the smoothies at age nine and now absolutely loves them. Be patient!
- Try making your own applesauce.
- Have your child pick out a different fruit for the family to try.
- Have a color challenge, where you mark a chart with each different color fruit served throughout the week.
- Use small cookie cutters or a melon baller to cut fruit into cute shapes.
- Offer dips such as guacamole or hummus to go along with veggies.
- Try preparing an unpopular fruit or veggie in a different way. If raw carrots don't fly, try steamed. If steamed broccoli isn't your child's cup of tea, try roasted.

- Provide seasoning and let your child sprinkle it atop the food. Try cinnamon on apples or in applesauce, garlic on roasted vegetables, and lemon juice on asparagus.
- Make a spinach or basil pesto to serve over whole-wheat pasta.

Patience, persistence, modeling, and exposure are the keys to increased fruit and vegetable intake. When you start to falter, let this helpful parent mantra be your guide: Serve a fruit and veggie, eat them yourself, then give yourself a pat on the back because your job is *done*! (Even if your child didn't eat it, you did your job by offering.)

2. Vegetable Haters

Like Picky Produce Eaters, Vegetable Haters balk at anything green, though they might enjoy fruit. Try these tips for getting them to enjoy eating more vegetables:

- Buy vegetables often. Cook vegetables often. Eat vegetables yourself often.
- Serve a tiny portion to your child at least once a day, without pressure.
- Ask your child to "kiss" the vegetable, smell it, or taste it with his tongue.
- If your child is the gagging and dramatic type, give him an out—either he doesn't need to put the whole thing in his mouth, or he can spit it out in a napkin.
- Keep trying. It can take at least a dozen times for an older toddler or child to accept a new food. Try all kinds—plain, flavored, roasted, in soups, in salads, with dip, etc.
- Don't worry about the actual amount of vegetables being consumed. Instead, throw your energy into making them

delicious and offering them often. Focus on *your* job: the preparing and the offering. Let your children be in charge of their job: the eating.

- Be positive and do not force.

3. Real Chicken Refusers

Real Chicken Refusers will eat only a certain kind of chicken—typically, breaded and deep-fried and *not* prepared at home (from scratch). Acceptable chicken is probably either from a restaurant or from a box, because kids like the consistency, taste, and appearance of these corporate-made foods. Try the following steps to convert a Real Chicken Refuser:

- Set a frequency limit on kid-friendly chicken—perhaps half as often as you're presently letting your child eat it.
- Cook "real" chicken at home. See the recipe section (chapter 15) for a few suggestions. Remember: your job is to serve the chicken, not to force your child to eat it.
- If your child asks, explain why he can't have fried chicken tenders all the time (for example, they're a once-in-a-while option and not good for every day).

4. White-Food Fans

Some kids want to eat only foods made with white flour (bread, pasta, crackers, and so on)—foods that are less nutritious than those made with whole grains. You can convert a White-Food Fan into a Fiber Imbiber slowly or quickly, and in all categories or just a few. Choose some of the strategies below to start with:

- Keep using white bread in sandwiches at lunch, but buy whole-wheat bread and use it to make French toast.
- Make pancakes using half regular flour and half whole-wheat flour. You can also try making pancakes with oatmeal.
- Offer toasted whole-wheat bread with yummy toppings or as cinnamon toast.
- Although your child may not immediately accept the homemade version of his favorite chicken tenders, involve him in preparing and serving them and after a few attempts he should accept and enjoy his new creation.
- Keep the white bread, but convert other food "categories" to higher-fiber alternatives—for example, switch your low-fiber cereal to a higher-fiber option.
- One popular strategy is to make *half* your grains *whole*. To accomplish this, think of all the grain-based products your family eats, such as pasta, bread, cold cereal, hot cereal, granola bars, pretzels, and crackers. Using this strategy, your family might choose to keep eating standard white pasta, but switch to a new whole-grain cereal and whole-grain crackers. (A whole-grain food will have an ingredient list that starts with "100 percent whole-wheat flour" or simply "oats" rather than the generic "enriched flour.")
- Consider a "washout period" for white bread—just stop buying it completely, and a very young child will forget about it fairly quickly (usually in a week or two).
- For very young children, you don't need to explain much. Just change your buying habits at the grocery store. When my kids were very young and would ask about a certain brand that I wanted to stop buying, I'd tell them that the store had been out of it.

BETH'S GROCERY GUIDE

Start at the Store

If your child demands only sugar cereals, for example, and you'd like him to branch out, the first step is to *stop buying them*! Have a two-week washout period. Or buy one box and let your child know that he will be able to eat it only once per week (or weekends only) instead of his current daily habit. Remember: you (the parent) are in charge!

- Make muffins/pancakes/waffles at home using half whole-wheat flour, and freeze the extras to have on hand for busy days.
- Some whole-wheat bread is admittedly not very tasty. Beth tried quite a few varieties before settling on two delicious brands that she and her two kids like. Make sure you actually *enjoy* the bread you're serving.

5. Backward Eaters

Most forms of picky eating boil down to what I call "backward eating." The Backward Eater truly desires the manufactured, processed version rather than the real, natural version, as in the following examples:

- Frozen breaded chicken nuggets (instead of real chicken)
- Fruit gummies (instead of fruit)
- Boxed macaroni and cheese (instead of homemade)
- The kids' meal from a restaurant (rather than the homemade version)
- Fake-colored sugar cereal (instead of a plainer version)

You need to understand that in the Backward Eater's mind, this "favorite" (but backward) item is the gold standard to which all other foods are compared. The "real" version doesn't measure up.

Unfortunately, the first time a child tries such a highly processed food, she may get hooked. Believe me, millions of dollars went into making that boxed mac and cheese exactly what children prefer. "Backward" favorites are usually both highly processed *and* marketed specifically to children.

The good news: backward eating is a problem only if a favorite food displaces the real or healthier version of that food. For example, a backward eater might love breaded, fried restaurant chicken tenders but refuse real chicken cooked at home. This is different than if a child begs for your homemade marinara sauce or homemade pizza—this is not backward eating. If a child loves fresh apples to the exclusion of all other fruit, I don't see this as a problem either; it's not backward eating.

Converting a Backward Eater usually requires reduced exposure, time, consistency, and home cooking.

Reduced Exposure

We know that children can develop brand loyalty at a very young age, even as toddlers. If my child was stuck on a certain boxed mac and cheese brand and I wanted to kick that habit, I would first reduce the exposure to the brand. If I had my child with me at the grocery store, I would completely avoid the boxed pasta aisle, or I would shop at a grocery store that didn't carry the brand. I would make foods completely unrelated to their favorite mac and cheese. I would understand that my child loves the bright orange color and specific taste of that brand's product. I would also understand that it would be very difficult to replicate this color and taste in a homemade version. Rather than trying, I would make chicken and plain pasta! Luckily, young children have short memory spans, so they soon forget about the favorite.

Time

Changing habits takes time, so be patient and give the hoped-for new behavior a few months to take effect.

Consistency

If I had a child who was "addicted" (just to simplify the terminology) to a drive-through kids' meal, I would minimize the exposure over time, as suggested above. But that's hard to maintain. The more frazzled and busy I got, the greater the chance I would resort to the drive-through, just to make my life easier. It's very important to try to be consistent in offering your healthier desired alternative to the favorite food, even if it's not as convenient for you.

Home Cooking

Rarely do parents complain that all their child wants to eat is homemade baked chicken. The unhealthy backward-eating favorite is generally a food made by a corporation, not in one's own kitchen. Hence, the healthier alternative is generally homemade. Please see the recipe section (chapter 15) for easy homemade versions of several traditional kid favorites.

Most kids will have some degree of pickiness before age five; it's a totally normal and expected phase. Though you can't change a picky eater, you can change your response to him. Don't cater to your picky eater; instead, make and serve one meal from which everyone chooses. Don't make any member of the family a special meal. Do keep offering fruits and vegetables, and consider your job done when you've put them on the table. Remember: your job is to provide a variety of foods, and your child's job is to decide whether to eat them. With patience, persistence, modeling, and time, you *can* convert a picky eater to one who loves to eat lots of different types of yummy, health-enhancing food!

Remember This

- Serve one meal only, from which everyone chooses and eats.
- Model healthy eating.
- Have lots of fruits and vegetables available, in child-accessible forms (washed, peeled, and cut).
- Live by the dictum that fruits and veggies rule: "All fruits, all vegetables, all forms." Try them steamed, roasted, in soups, in smoothies, with dips, and more!
- Remember and repeat the parent mantra: "Serve a fruit and veggie! Eat it myself! Now my job is done! (Even if my child didn't eat it, I did my job by offering.)"
- It is fine to encourage trying new foods, but do not force your child to swallow something he is truly anxious about eating.
- It can take six to twelve months of intervention before a dedicated picky eater is converted to a wider variety of food.

PART FOUR

Recipes

15.

Nutritious and Delicious Recipes

Baby Food

For all the baby-food recipes listed here, good equipment choices for pureeing include a high-powered blender, an immersion blender, a regular or mini-food processor, and any of the many baby-food blending gadgets available.

Baby-Food Broccoli

FOUNDATION FOOD: Green Vegetables

Makes enough to fill one ice-cube tray

2 bunches of broccoli
2 tablespoons water (reserved from cooking)
Tiny pinch of kosher salt (optional)

Cut off (and discard) the broccoli stems, and wash the crowns. Cook the broccoli 3 to 4 minutes or until tender, using one of these methods: arrange the broccoli in a steamer basket set over boiling water in a pot on the stove, then cover the pot; *or* place it in boiling water (you can salt the water if you prefer), then cool immediately in ice water; *or* steam it in a little water in the microwave. Reserve the cooking water. Place the cooked broccoli in a high-powered blender, along with 2 tablespoons reserved cooking water. Blend on high until pureed. After tasting, add a tiny pinch of kosher salt if desired (maybe ⅛ teaspoon) and blend again, then taste again. Divide the pureed broccoli equally across an ice-cube tray. Cool the filled tray to room temperature and then freeze it. When the puree is solid, transfer the cubes into a freezer-safe container.

Baby-Food Carrots

FOUNDATION FOOD: Even though carrots aren't one of the Eleven Foundation Foods, they are super-healthy and can easily be mixed with almost any green vegetable, chicken, or legume.

I use bunches of organic carrots (preferably with the greens attached for freshness, though the greens aren't used in cooking), and I keep the skin on the carrots because I don't like peeling them. Dr. Tanya peels her carrots first. Your choice, obviously! You can also use bagged baby carrots, but give them a quick wash first. Make tons of extra baby-food carrots to mix with chicken or green veggies.

Makes enough to fill two ice-cube trays

2 large bunches of fresh carrots
2 to 3 tablespoons water (reserved from cooking)

Cut off and discard the ends of the carrots. Wash the carrots (and peel them if desired). Cut each carrot into three to four pieces. Steam the carrots until tender (using one of the methods described on page 270), reserving the cooking water. Transfer the cooked chunks to a high-powered blender, along with 2 to 3 tablespoons reserved cooking water, and puree. Pour the mixture into an ice-cube tray, cool the filled tray to room temperature, and freeze it. When the puree is solid, transfer the cubes into a freezer-safe container.

Baby-Food Strawberries

FOUNDATION FOOD: Berries

If fresh strawberries aren't in season, use frozen! You can simply defrost them before blending as directed below. This recipe can also be used for other berries and almost any other fruit.

Makes enough to fill half of an ice-cube tray

1 pint strawberries
1 tablespoon water

Wash berries well. Cut them into halves or thirds and transfer them to a blender or food processor. Add the water and blend to the desired consistency, adding more water if needed.

Baby-Food Eggs

FOUNDATION FOOD: Eggs

Dr. Tanya makes a bunch of hard-boiled eggs and keeps them in the refrigerator for a few days because her older boys like them. She pureed one and gave it to her baby as an experiment—another hit!

1 egg makes about 2 baby-size servings

1 to 2 hard-boiled eggs
1 teaspoon water or breast milk
Tiny pinch of salt if desired

Put the hard-boiled eggs in a baby-food processor. Add water and blend to the desired consistency, adding more water (or breast milk) if needed. This puree will keep for two to three days in the refrigerator.

Baby-Food Chicken

 **FOUNDATION FOOD: Chicken**

I've experimented making chicken two ways: roasting and poaching. Both turn out fine, but the flavor of the roasted chicken is a little better. If you're roasting chicken for your family, make a few extra pieces for your baby! Any cut is fine, but I prefer thighs or drumsticks for very young eaters, because they don't dry out as easily. You can also use boneless, skinless chicken breast, but be careful not to overcook it and thus dry it out. I use my mini–food processor to grind the chicken in seconds.

Makes enough to fill one ice-cube tray

A few pieces of bone-in, skin-on chicken
½ teaspoon olive oil (for roasting)
⅛ to ¼ teaspoon salt, optional
Pureed cooked carrots, pureed cooked sweet potato, or any other pureed cooked veggie (optional)

FOR ROASTING: Preheat the oven to 425°F. Line a baking sheet with foil. Rub the chicken with a little olive oil and sprinkle with the salt, if desired. Roast about 20 minutes, or until the internal temperature of the chicken reaches 165°F.

FOR STOVETOP POACHING: Place the chicken in a pot and cover it with 2 inches of water above the chicken. Bring the pot to a boil and then reduce to simmer. Simmer the chicken, covered, about 20 minutes, or until its internal temperature reaches 165°F. Reserve the cooking liquid.

FOR BOTH: After the chicken is cooked, let it cool slightly so that it's easy to handle. Remove the skin and pull the meat off the bones. Put the meat into a mini–food processor and add 1 tablespoon cooking liquid (use chicken broth or water if you don't have any liquid left). Chop or grind the chicken until it's very small. You can store the chicken alone or mixed with the pureed vegetables. Spoon whichever combination of purees you like into an ice-cube tray and freeze it. When the puree is solid, transfer the cubes into a freezer-safe container.

Baby-Food Sweet Potatoes

FOUNDATION FOOD: Again, though not a member of the Eleven Foundation Foods, sweet potatoes are nutritious and delicious! Like carrots, they are excellent for mixing with green veggies, chicken, and beans.

Makes enough to fill one ice-cube tray

3 large sweet potatoes

Preheat the oven to 400°F. Wash the potatoes and poke holes in them. Place the potatoes on a foil-lined baking sheet and bake them for 60 minutes, or until tender. After the sweet potatoes have cooled, remove (and discard) the skins and mash the pulp well. Add water if needed to thin the mash. Spoon the mash into an ice-cube tray and freeze it. When the mash is solid, transfer the cubes into a freezer-safe container.

Sweet Summer Corn and Cauliflower

 **FOUNDATION FOOD: Green Vegetables**

I put cauliflower in the category of green vegetables (because to me it is just like broccoli) even though it's typically white. Actually, you can find green Romanesco and even purple cauliflower at some farmers' markets and stores. Romanesco and purple cauliflower are two of my favorites!

I made corn on the cob for my kids one summer night and wanted to try it as a baby food. The corn alone I found a little too sweet and pasty, so I decided to try mixing it with steamed cauliflower. The corn and cauliflower combo tastes great!

Makes enough to fill one ice-cube tray

2 to 3 ears corn on the cob
2 tablespoons sugar
1 head cauliflower, cut into florets
⅛ to ¼ teaspoon salt (optional)

FOR THE CORN: Bring a large pot of water plus the sugar to a boil. Add the corn and boil, covered, for 5 minutes. Cool and remove the corn from the cob. Reserve ¼ cup cooking water.

FOR THE CAULIFLOWER: Steam cauliflower florets until tender.

Put the cooked corn, cooked cauliflower, and about ¼ cup cooking water into the blender. Blend until pureed, adding extra water if needed. After tasting, add the salt if desired; blend again to mix the salt in well. Pour the vegetable puree into an ice-cube tray, cool to room temperature, and freeze. When the puree is solid, transfer the cubes into a freezer-safe container.

Purple Oatmeal

FOUNDATION FOODS: Whole Grains, Prunes

Oatmeal is a healthy way to start your baby's day. The prunes help prevent and even treat your baby's constipation, and the fruit also adds a little sweetness to the cereal. It's easy to get into a routine of adding prunes to your baby's breakfast. All three of Dr. Tanya's boys loved Purple Oatmeal when they were young.

Makes 1 serving; easily doubled

Baby oatmeal cereal
Baby-food prunes

Make a 1-ounce serving (or more) of baby oatmeal cereal according to package directions. For every ounce of cooked oatmeal, add 1 to 2 teaspoons baby-food prunes.

Peanut Butter Oatmeal

FOUNDATION FOODS: Whole Grains, Nuts

Please read chapter 8 on food allergies and check with your pediatrician before serving this to your baby if you have any concerns about food allergies. Make sure the consistency is very thin so that your baby can easily handle it.

Makes 1 serving; easily doubled

Baby oatmeal cereal
Creamy peanut butter

Make a 1-ounce serving (or more) of baby oatmeal cereal according to package directions. For every ounce of cooked oatmeal, add 1 teaspoon peanut butter. Add more liquid if needed to decrease stickiness.

Make-Ahead Breakfast Burritos

FOUNDATION FOODS: Eggs, Whole Grains, Green Vegetables, Cheese, Avocados

You can add any vegetables you like to this dish, or keep it simple if your child prefers a plainer egg dish. These burritos make a perfect breakfast for child *and* parent: you can give the child all the components separately, and you can compose a traditional burrito for yourself. Since you assemble everything ahead of time, this recipe is a good choice for busy days.

Makes 4 servings

6 eggs
¼ cup milk
¼ teaspoon salt, or to taste
¼ teaspoon ground black pepper, or to taste
2 tablespoons unsalted butter
¼ cup chopped green bell pepper
½ cup shredded cheese
4 whole-wheat tortillas
1 avocado, chopped (optional)

Crack the eggs into a medium bowl and beat with a fork until well blended. Add the milk, salt, and pepper, and mix well. In a nonstick skillet over medium heat, melt the butter. Sauté the chopped green bell pepper in the butter for 3 to 4 minutes. Add the egg mixture and cook, gently moving the eggs in the skillet using a wooden spoon, until the eggs are softly scrambled. Add the cheese and gently stir it in. Remove the pan from the heat and let the contents cool to room temperature. Transfer the cooked egg mixture to a covered container and refrigerate, unless you plan to serve the burritos immediately.

To assemble (whether immediately, later in the day, or the next day), heat the tortillas in the microwave for 30 seconds, or on a hot griddle or skillet for about a minute per side. Fill each tortilla with a strip of egg mixture and chopped avocado and roll them up. If the filling is cold, cook the burrito until hot.

Fabulous French Toast

FOUNDATION FOODS: Whole Grains, Milk, Eggs

I suggest making extra pieces of this delicious French toast so that you can have leftovers at breakfast—or as a snack—the next day. The vanilla creamer I use has only four ingredients; some brands have extremely long ingredient lists and should be avoided. You could instead add a tiny amount of vanilla extract—maybe ⅛ teaspoon.

Makes 4 servings

4 eggs
2 to 3 tablespoons milk
1 tablespoon natural vanilla creamer (optional)
Pinch of cinnamon
4 slices 100 percent whole-wheat bread

Preheat a nonstick griddle or griddle pan using medium heat. Crack the eggs into a bowl and add the milk, creamer (if using), and cinnamon. Beat well by hand. Dip the bread into the mixture, letting the excess drip off. Cook each side 2 to 4 minutes, or until golden.

Yogurt Breakfast Buffet

 **FOUNDATION FOODS: Yogurt, Whole Grains, Nuts, Berries**

This recipe is fun for older toddlers and preschoolers because they can choose their mix-ins and even help layer the ingredients to make a parfait. Serve the parfait in clear bowls or cups so that kids can see the layers. Parents and children can enjoy this breakfast together.

The number of servings is variable

Plain or vanilla Greek or regular yogurt
Fresh or thawed frozen berries, washed and chopped
Finely chopped nuts such as walnuts
Crushed graham crackers (optional)
Honey or fruit preserves (optional)

Set out ingredients in medium-size bowls and let each child pick which items she wants. Together, layer each item into small bowls or cups.

Egg Cups

FOUNDATION FOODS: Eggs, Milk, Green Vegetables, Cheese

This dish is amazing, because kids can feed themselves; the muffin-shape eggs are easy to handle. You can make them in mini-muffin pans or standard muffin pans, in many different variations, including with veggies. Don't remove them from the oven until you see the tops puff up. Thanks to Amy G. for the recipe inspiration.

Makes about 12 mini or 6 regular servings

1 cup frozen shredded potatoes, slightly thawed
8 eggs
3 tablespoons milk
Pinch of salt
Pinch of ground black pepper
Optional: **Finely chopped broccoli, red or green bell pepper, tomato, onion, or almost any vegetable; shredded cheese; diced ham or cooked turkey bacon or cooked turkey sausage**

Preheat the oven to 350°F. Prepare a muffin pan (either mini-muffin or standard) by spraying *very well* with nonstick cooking spray. Nest 1 to 2 tablespoons of the potatoes in the bottom of each muffin well. (The amount of potato will vary depending on which pan you're using.) Bake just the potatoes for about 10 minutes. While those are baking, crack the eggs into a large glass measuring cup; add the milk, salt, and pepper to the eggs and whisk well.

Although the vegetables don't need to be precooked, they will taste better if you lightly sauté them first. To sauté, heat 2 teaspoons of oil in a skillet over medium heat, then add the vegetables and cook for about 5 minutes, stirring occasionally.

Add vegetables (if using) into egg mixture. Pour the egg mixture over the partially cooked potatoes, until each well is about two-thirds full. Bake 15 to 20 minutes, or until the tops puff up.

Whole-Wheat Bursting-with-Blueberry Muffins

FOUNDATION FOODS: Berries, Whole Grains, Milk, Eggs

Having experimented with many different muffin recipes, I finally created this tender, yummy whole-wheat muffin. In the end I combined a *Gourmet* magazine recipe with a blueberry jam technique from America's Test Kitchen, then swapped out milk for buttermilk because I like the taste and texture it provides. Do not use regular whole-wheat flour; you must use whole-wheat pastry flour for best results.

Makes 12 muffins

2½ cups blueberries, fresh or thawed frozen (divided)
½ cup sugar (divided)
1¾ cups whole-wheat pastry flour
2 teaspoons baking powder
¾ teaspoon salt
1 teaspoon grated lemon zest
5 tablespoons unsalted butter, melted
½ cup buttermilk
1 large egg, beaten with fork

Preheat the oven to 375°F and put the rack in the lower-middle oven. Fill a standard muffin pan with paper liners.

Combine 1 cup blueberries and 1 tablespoon sugar in a small saucepan. Cook on medium-low heat and mash the berries with a potato masher or a fork. Once the berries start breaking down, let them simmer 5 minutes. Remove the pan from the heat and let the "jam" cool for a few minutes.

In a large bowl, combine the flour, remaining sugar, baking powder, and salt with a whisk. Add the lemon zest and whisk again. In a separate small bowl, combine the melted butter, buttermilk, and egg, and whisk well. Make a well in the dry-ingredients bowl. Add the wet ingredients to the dry ingredients and gently fold together with a rubber spatula, until the ingredients are just combined. (Do not overmix.) The batter will be lumpy. Add the remaining 1½ cups berries and gently fold to combine. Add the cooled berry jam and fold it in gently. You don't want to thoroughly blend the mixture—there should be streaks of both yellow batter and blue jam.

Use a scoop to fill the muffin cups about two-thirds full. Bake for 20 minutes, or until a toothpick inserted in the center has no batter clinging to it when removed. Cool muffins in the pan 5 minutes, then remove them to a rack to finish cooling.

Chocolate Chip Muffins

 **FOUNDATION FOODS: Whole Grains, Milk, Eggs**

You can serve these muffins at breakfast, for snack, or for a treat. They use an equal combination of whole-wheat and regular flour, boosting the nutrients and fiber (whole-wheat), but also keeping the muffins tender (regular).

Makes 24 mini-muffins

1 cup whole-wheat pastry flour
1 cup all-purpose flour
¼ cup buttermilk + ¼ cup half-and-half (or ½ cup of either, alone)
½ cup (1 stick) unsalted butter, at room temperature
1 cup sugar
2 teaspoons baking powder
½ teaspoon salt
1 teaspoon vanilla extract
½ teaspoon almond extract
2 large eggs, cracked into a bowl and whisked
1 cup mini-chocolate chips

Preheat the oven to 350°F. Line a mini-muffin pan with paper liners. Put both flours into a small bowl and stir together; set aside. Mix the buttermilk and half-and-half together; set aside. In a large mixing bowl, combine the butter, sugar, baking powder, salt, vanilla extract, and almond extract. (Yes, it's correct to add the baking powder and salt in this step.) Beat with an electric or stand mixer until fluffy, about 3 to 4 minutes. Scrape down the sides of the bowl with a rubber spatula. Add the eggs and beat at medium speed about 1 to 2 minutes, until combined. Scrape down the bowl again. Add the buttermilk mixture, hand-stirring with the rubber spatula until well combined. Add the flour, gently folding it in until just combined; this should take less than 1 minute. (Do not overmix!) Fold in the chocolate chips until evenly distributed.

Use a small cookie scoop to gently place balls of batter in each mini-muffin liner. Bake 10 to 12 minutes, then check. The muffins are done when a toothpick inserted in the center comes out clean. If you need to keep the muffins in longer, check each minute to prevent overbaking. Cool in the pan for 5 minutes, then transfer to a wire rack to cool completely.

Pizza

FOUNDATION FOODS: Green Vegetables, Cheese

I like to use a frozen plain pizza crust for this recipe because it's very easy. Even with that shortcut, the final product (otherwise homemade) has far fewer ingredients and preservatives than a frozen premade pizza.

Makes 4 to 6 servings

1 frozen plain pizza crust (Trader Joe's sells frozen plain pizza crusts)

½ cup refrigerated or jarred pizza sauce

1 cup shredded mozzarella cheese

Green veggie toppings of choice, such as cut green bell peppers or broccoli

Preheat the oven to 425°F, or whatever temperature the pizza crust packaging recommends. Prepare a pizza pan according to the directions on the packaging and lay the crust on it. Pour the sauce on the crust and let any older children spread it around. Sprinkle the cheese on the pizza—another job that the kids can help with—and distribute the green veggies evenly. Bake the pizza according to the pizza crust packaging directions.

Stovetop Macaroni and Cheese

 **FOUNDATION FOODS: Milk, Cheese**

Makes 4 servings

1 cup dry elbow macaroni
1 cup milk (preferably whole or 2 percent)
1 tablespoon cornstarch
¼ teaspoon dry mustard powder
¼ teaspoon salt
⅛ teaspoon ground black pepper
1 cup shredded cheese (ideally half jack, half cheddar, but you can also use all cheddar)

Cook the pasta according to package directions. Combine the milk and the cornstarch in a small saucepan and mix well with a whisk, getting rid of any clumps. Add mustard powder, salt, and pepper, and mix again. Cook over medium heat, stirring constantly. When the mixture starts to simmer, keep stirring; let it simmer 1 minute. Remove the pan from the heat and stir in the cheese. Add the cooked pasta to the cheese sauce and stir well.

Breaded Chicken Drumsticks

 **FOUNDATION FOODS: Chicken, Yogurt**

I saw this recipe on *Bon Appétit's* Twitter feed and decided to try it. It was a great hit—the drumsticks turned out crispy and crunchy—so I've adapted it here. For small children, just pull the meat off the bones and serve in small pieces.

Makes about 6 servings

½ cup plain yogurt (preferably 2 percent)
2 tablespoons jarred Dijon mustard
1 cup panko bread crumbs
1 teaspoon kosher salt
1 teaspoon black pepper
1 pack skin-on chicken drumsticks (about 6 drumsticks)

Preheat the oven to 425°F. Set a wire rack on top of a cookie sheet. Mix the yogurt and mustard together in a medium bowl. In a large resealable plastic bag, mix the panko, salt, and pepper. Using your fingers, coat the chicken pieces with the yogurt mixture, then place all the chicken pieces into the bag, seal it, and shake well to coat with bread crumbs. (You can use a disposable kitchen glove to handle the chicken, if you like.) Place the coated chicken on the wire rack for cooking. Bake until the coating browns nicely, about 40 to 50 minutes. Remove from the oven and let sit 5 minutes before serving.

Super-Quick Deconstructed Salad Bar

 **FOUNDATION FOODS: Citrus, Green Vegetables, Chicken**

I love serving a deconstructed salad bar for lunch or dinner. Preschool kids can handle it, and some older toddlers as well. The possibilities are endless, but here is an Asian chicken salad variation inspired by a recipe from the Halos mandarins website. The key is serving every item in a little bowl, just as at a restaurant salad bar. I use time-savers such as prebagged organic lettuce, but you can certainly chop your own. If I'm using just a small amount of an ingredient like purple cabbage, I'll often buy it from a grocery store salad bar. You don't have to cook a chicken specially for this recipe: use leftover chicken or a store-bought rotisserie chicken.

The number of servings is variable

1 bag romaine lettuce
1 cup shredded purple cabbage
1 to 2 cups mandarin or tangerine segments (fresh, not canned)
1 cup finely diced carrots
2 cups cooked chicken in small pieces
2 green onions, finely diced
Crunchy noodle toppings or wonton strips (optional)
Asian dressing of your choice

Wash the bagged lettuce well. Place all remaining ingredients in separate small bowls and serve them salad-bar style.

Black Bean Quesadillas

 **FOUNDATION FOODS: Beans, Whole Grains, Cheese, Green Vegetables**

This recipe is very easy, super-healthy, and filled with fiber and protein. I like it because if the kids don't care for the bell peppers you can easily omit them from theirs but add them to yours for the extra flavor. (The peppers really do make the dish much more complex and delicious.) I adapted this dish from a recipe created by Deborah Turobiner; you can find her recipes at myyummyinyourtummy.blogspot.com.

Don't be tempted to skip toasting the tortillas; they improve in taste and texture in that step.

Makes 2 to 4 servings

2 whole-wheat tortillas
1 teaspoon olive or canola oil
½ cup frozen bell pepper strips (any color, or mixed)
Pinch of salt
Pinch of ground black pepper
1 cup shredded mozzarella or jack cheese
½ cup black beans, drained

On a griddle or in a large nonstick pan over medium heat, cook each tortilla, turning once, for 2 to 4 minutes, or until they start to crisp. Remove the griddle from the heat but leave the tortillas on it. Add 1 teaspoon oil to a small saucepan (preheated over medium heat) and let the oil heat up. Add the bell peppers to the saucepan and sauté, stirring occasionally, until they're soft and heated through, about 6 to 10 minutes. Season the peppers with salt and pepper. Sprinkle cheese atop half of each crisped tortilla; then add beans and peppers. Return the griddle to the heat and let the fillings heat through, 1 to 2 more minutes; then fold the tortillas in half.

Turkey Avocado Wrap

 **FOUNDATION FOODS: Whole Grains, Avocados, Cheese**

Makes 1 serving; can easily be multiplied

1 whole-grain tortilla or corn tortilla
2 ounces sliced nitrate-free deli turkey
¼ to ½ avocado, mashed or sliced
2 ounces provolone cheese, sliced
Drizzle of store-bought or homemade ranch dressing (optional)

Lay out the tortilla and layer turkey, avocado, and cheese on top. Drizzle dressing over ingredients if desired. Roll the wrap up tightly to serve.

Crispy Baked Fish Sticks

FOUNDATION FOODS: Fish, Eggs

This recipe is adapted from one created by chef Patti Anastasia, a colleague of mine. Patti adapted it from a Rachael Ray recipe.

Makes 4 servings

2 tablespoons vegetable oil

¾ to 1 pound fresh or thawed frozen boneless cod or halibut fillets

1½ to 2 teaspoons salt (divided)

½ teaspoon ground black pepper

1 cup all-purpose flour

3 large eggs

1 cup panko bread crumbs

¼ teaspoon ground cayenne pepper (it doesn't make them spicy!)

Spread the vegetable oil on a baking sheet. Preheat the oven to 450°F. Place the baking sheet in the upper third of the oven. Cut the fish fillets into strips about 1 inch wide. In a shallow bowl, mix 1 teaspoon salt and the black pepper into the flour, stirring to combine. Crack the eggs into a second shallow bowl and whisk them with a fork to blend whites and yolks. Place the panko in a third shallow bowl and add the cayenne pepper and an additional ½ to 1 teaspoon salt. Dip the fish in this order: flour, then eggs, then bread crumbs. Place breaded fish on the hot baking sheet. Bake 10 minutes, turning once in the middle. Set on a paper towel–lined plate for 2 minutes, then serve and enjoy!

Circle "French Fries"

FOUNDATION FOOD: Though not one of the Eleven Foundation Foods, potatoes are nutritious. They are excellent to serve alongside green veggies, chicken, and beans.

This quick go-to side dish, a more nutritious version of a kid favorite, is much healthier than fried potatoes. I make it in my toaster oven, which has a convection-bake option, but you can make it in a regular oven as well.

Makes 4 to 6 servings

6 to 10 yellow baby potatoes (the small, long kind)
⅓ cup canola oil
½ teaspoon kosher salt
¼ teaspoon ground black pepper

Preheat the oven to 400°F. Line a cookie sheet with parchment paper or foil. Wash the potatoes and trim a bit off each end. Slice the potatoes into ½- to ⅓-inch circles. Place all the rounds into a bowl and drizzle them with the canola oil. Sprinkle with the salt and pepper. Mix very well so that each round is coated evenly. Place the potato pieces (no overlapping) on the parchment- or foil-covered cookie sheet. Bake about 15 minutes; then stir the potatoes and cook them 10 to 15 minutes more, checking every 5 minutes for doneness. They should be tender inside and golden brown and crispy outside.

Lemon-Rosemary Roast Chicken

 **FOUNDATION FOOD: Chicken**

Ree Drummond, aka the Pioneer Woman, has a great roast lemon chicken recipe on her website that I've adapted here. I made it a faster dish by using chicken pieces rather than the whole bird. (Her recipe is available at thepioneerwoman.com if you prefer to cook a whole chicken.) After you put the chicken into the oven, you can forget about it for 30 minutes. This is mostly hands-off cooking, which makes it a great choice for busy parents. Do *not* use boneless, skinless meat in this recipe.

Makes 4 to 6 servings

3 to 4 chicken breasts, skin-on, bone-in (or an entire cut-up chicken, or 8 thighs, or a combination)
½ cup (1 stick) unsalted butter, at room temperature
1 to 2 tablespoons grated lemon zest
1 sprig rosemary, chopped
¼ teaspoon salt
⅛ teaspoon ground black pepper

Preheat the oven to 450°F. Pat the chicken dry using paper towels. In a small bowl, combine the softened butter, lemon zest, rosemary, salt, and pepper. Smear the butter mixture all over the top (skin side) of the chicken, coating the meat well. Place the chicken pieces skin-side up in an oven-safe skillet (not nonstick). Roast 30 minutes, then check the meat's internal temperature. Chicken is done when it reaches 165°F. If the chicken needs more time, check it every

5 minutes until it reaches the desired internal temperature. After removing the pan carefully from the oven, cover it loosely with foil and let the dish rest 10 minutes before serving.

Sautéed Green Beans (or Other Veggies)

FOUNDATION FOOD: Green Vegetables

My kids like their vegetables on the plainer side, but I prefer added flavor. Here is an easy way everyone can eat the veggies to their liking. On busy weeknights I often use prebagged vegetables from the grocery store. Green beans, broccoli, and sugar snap peas are among the vegetables available already cut and washed.

The number of servings is variable

12 to 16 ounces of your vegetable of choice, such as green beans, broccoli, or sugar snap peas, washed and trimmed
1 to 2 tablespoons olive oil and/or butter
1 to 2 cloves garlic (fresh or frozen), minced
¼ to ½ teaspoon salt (optional)
¼ teaspoon ground black pepper (optional)
½ to 1 teaspoon lemon juice

Steam veggies until they're crisp-tender and set them aside. (I use a microwave steamer, but you can also steam vegetables above simmering water, using a colander or a metal steamer, with the pot loosely covered.) Put the oil and/or butter in a small saucepan over medium heat. Add the garlic and cook, stirring, for 1 to 2 minutes. Throw in whatever vegetable you've chosen and stir again. Add salt, pepper, and lemon juice if desired.

Robin's Lentil Soup

 **FOUNDATION FOOD: Lentils**

My neighbor Robin used to make this soup for her infant granddaughter. When the baby first started solids, Robin mashed the lentils very well to make the soup more manageable. Now that the baby is older, everyone can eat from the same recipe. When I make this soup, I often use short-cut products such as precooked steamed lentils and a prechopped container of mirepoix. If you have more time, of course you can prep and chop everything yourself. The result is easy, healthy, and delicious!

Makes 4 to 6 servings

2 tablespoons olive or canola oil
1 14.5-ounce container mirepoix (or ½ cup each chopped onions, celery, and carrots)
2 cubes frozen garlic, or 2 teaspoons chopped fresh garlic
1 17.6-ounce package ready-to-eat lentils (or 2 to 3 cups cooked lentils prepared according to package directions)
2 cups low-sodium chicken broth or vegetable broth
Pinch of salt (optional)
Pinch of ground black pepper (optional)

Heat the olive or canola oil in a large pot over medium heat. Add the mirepoix and cook 6 to 8 minutes, until soft. Add the garlic and cook an additional 30 seconds, stirring frequently so that the garlic does not burn. Add the lentils and chicken or vegetable broth. Stir the soup well, cover, and simmer 30 minutes. Mash the lentils with a potato masher, then cook another 10 minutes. Season with salt and pepper if desired.

Easy Chicken Tenders

 **FOUNDATION FOOD: Chicken**

You can prepare this dish entirely on the stovetop; however, many beginning cooks find that by the time the chicken is cooked through, they've burned the outside. Finishing the chicken in the oven allows even and easy cooking.

Makes 4 servings

1 pound boneless, skinless chicken tenders
¼ cup flour
Pinch of salt
Pinch of ground black pepper
2 tablespoons olive or canola oil (divided)

If you have time, take the chicken out of the refrigerator and let it come to room temperature for 15 to 20 minutes. Preheat the oven to 350°F. Combine the flour, salt, and pepper in a large resealable plastic bag or large bowl. Add the chicken tenders to the flour mixture and stir to coat lightly.

Place a large oven-safe skillet (*not* nonstick) over medium-high heat. When the pan is hot, add 1 tablespoon oil and heat it until shimmering. Add the chicken in a single layer, with space between each piece. (You may have to cook it in two batches, adding oil again before the second.) Do not move the chicken—let it cook in the pan for 2 to 3 minutes. It should turn a nice golden brown. Flip the chicken over and let the other side brown for 2 to 3 minutes. If chicken is not cooked through entirely (at 165°F), finish it by baking it in the oven another 5 minutes.

Note: You can use regular chicken breasts for this recipe as well. For bigger chicken breasts, you'll definitely benefit from browning on the stovetop and then finishing in the oven.

Salmon Two Ways

Both of these recipes are baked; however, you can also barbecue salmon or cook it right on the stovetop.

Simple Salmon

 **FOUNDATION FOOD: Fish**

Makes 3 to 4 servings

2 6-ounce salmon fillets, skin removed

2 tablespoons olive oil

¼ teaspoon salt

⅛ teaspoon ground black pepper

Preheat the oven to 400°F. Cover a baking sheet with nonstick cooking spray, or top the baking sheet with parchment paper to ease cleanup. Coat the salmon with olive oil—top, bottom, and sides. Sprinkle the salt and pepper on both sides of the salmon. Put the salmon skin-side down on the baking sheet. Place in the oven and bake 12 to 14 minutes or until your desired level of doneness. To test for doneness, cut into the center of a piece; it should be light pink and appear done.

Pesto Salmon

FOUNDATION FOOD: Fish

Makes 3 to 4 servings

2 6-ounce salmon fillets, skin removed
2 tablespoons fresh refrigerated pesto
2 tablespoons unsalted butter, at room temperature

Preheat the oven to 400°F. Cover a baking sheet with nonstick cooking spray, or top the baking sheet with parchment paper to ease cleanup. Place the salmon skin-side down on the baking sheet. In small bowl, combine the pesto and butter into a paste. Dot the pesto atop the salmon so that the fish is completely coated on top. You may use extra for more flavor if desired. Bake the fish 12 to 14 minutes or until your desired level of doneness. To test for doneness, cut into the center of a piece; it should be light pink and appear done.

Slow-Cooker Meals

A slow cooker, an electric appliance that cooks food at low temperatures for a long time, can be a busy parent's best friend! I'll often start a slow-cooker dinner in the morning or early afternoon, when the kids are occupied and I have more energy and time; later, when we're all tired out, the food is ready for us. As a double bonus, most slow-cooker food is extremely moist and tender, making it very kid-friendly. Cut or shred such food into tiny pieces for the youngest toddlers and even ten- to twelve-month-old babies.

Most foods cook best in a slow cooker without much liquid. You need no more than a cup of liquid for most dishes. You may find, when cooking meat in the slow cooker, that a quick brown on the stovetop beforehand adds layers of flavor and a deeper color to your finished dish.

Slow-Cooker Potato Leek Soup

 FOUNDATION FOOD: **Green Vegetables**

I adapted this recipe from Beth Hensperger, who has many yummy slow-cooker recipes in her books and on her website at bethhensperger.com. You can serve this pureed soup to babies, adults, and everyone in between! I use my high-powered blender to get a silky finish. Because leeks can be a pain to clean, I use prepared leeks from Trader Joe's; you can also use their frozen leeks. Use one leek per potato if you make this recipe smaller or larger.

Makes 4 to 6 servings

3 leeks, washed and thinly sliced; or the frozen equivalent, thawed

3 medium russet potatoes, peeled and diced

(continued)

3 to 4 cups water, vegetable broth, or chicken broth—enough to barely cover leeks and potatoes

½ teaspoon salt

¼ teaspoon ground white pepper

1 to 2 tablespoons unsalted butter, at room temperature

1 to 2 tablespoons heavy cream (optional)

Place the leeks and potatoes in the slow cooker. Add the water or broth to the pot, just to cover. Cover with the lid and cook the vegetables on low for 5 to 7 hours, until the potatoes are tender. Transfer in batches to a high-powered blender and puree. Add salt and white pepper. Add the butter and cream (if desired), and puree again. Taste for seasonings and add additional salt and/or pepper if desired.

Almond-Oat Granola Bars

 **FOUNDATION FOODS: Whole Grains, Nuts**

Makes 10 to 12 bars

1½ cup Marcona almonds or slivered regular almonds—no skin
¼ cup 100 percent-pure maple syrup
¼ cup packed light-brown sugar
2½ teaspoons vanilla
¼ teaspoon salt
¼ cup plus 1 tablespoon canola oil
2 cups old-fashioned oats

Preheat the oven to 300°F. Line a large rimmed baking sheet with a silicone baking mat or parchment paper. In a mini–food processor, pulse the almonds fifteen times. If not using a food processor, roughly chop the almonds. In a large bowl, whisk together the syrup, sugar, vanilla, salt, and oil. Add the oats and nuts and stir the mixture well, using a rubber spatula. Turn the dough out onto the cookie sheet. Using a stiff metal spatula, gently press the dough into a 9 × 13-inch rectangle. Try to make the dough even on the top and all sides. Bake uncovered for 15 minutes. Then cover with foil and bake another 15 minutes. Check the color: the dough should be a light golden brown and beginning to harden. Take the foil off and bake another 5 minutes uncovered. If granola is still very soft or not yet light golden brown, keep baking in 5-minute increments, checking each time. Let cool for 1 hour. When cool, gently break into pieces and store in an airtight container or resealable bag.

Berry Snack Bars

FOUNDATION FOODS: Berries, Whole Grains

Kids love supermarket cereal bars, but most such products are low-fiber filler foods with long ingredient lists. My inspiration comes from Ree Drummond, who uses strawberry preserves in her bars, but I wanted to use either fresh or frozen berries. I also changed to whole-wheat pastry flour instead of regular flour. The result is yummy. I can't stop eating these treats! Cut them into small bars and wrap in wax paper. They're great for breakfast, for snack, in school lunches, and even for dessert.

Makes 8 bars

8 tablespoons butter (divided), at room temperature and cut into 8 pieces
2 to 3 cups fresh or thawed frozen berries (half blueberries, half strawberries is best)
2 to 3 tablespoons granulated sugar
¾ cup whole-wheat pastry flour (*not* regular whole-wheat flour)
¾ cup old-fashioned oats
½ cup light-brown sugar (no need to pack it tightly)
½ teaspoon baking powder
¼ teaspoon salt

Preheat the oven to 375°F. Slice off 1 tablespoon butter and use it to grease an 8 × 8-inch glass or Pyrex baking dish. Place the berries and granulated sugar in a small saucepan over medium-low heat. They will need to cook down for about 15 to 20 minutes, until the mixture starts to look syrupy and most of the water has cooked out. Every so often, mash the berries down with a spoon. If you started with 3 cups, you should end up with about 1 cup; measurements do not need to be exact. Let the fruit cool 5 to 10 minutes.

In a medium bowl, combine the flour, oats, brown sugar, baking powder, and salt. Whisk to combine well and dissolve any large lumps of brown sugar. Add the remaining butter to the bowl and blend with a pastry blender (best choice), a large fork, or even a strong whisk. This step will take about 5 minutes. You want to gradually work the butter in, not stir it in. After about 5 minutes the dough will start to look well mixed but still crumbly. It's not a batter; it should remain crumbly. Put half the dough into the baking dish and press to evenly coat the bottom, plus about ¼ inch up the sides. Add more of the oat mixture if needed.

Spoon the fruit mixture onto the crust and use a small spatula to gently spread it. Carefully sprinkle the remaining oat mixture evenly over the fruit, and again very gently spread it if needed. Be careful to not mix the two layers.

Bake about 30 minutes, or until golden brown. Let cool, then cut right in the pan.

Berry Smoothie

FOUNDATION FOODS: Berries, Yogurt

I love using frozen berries when making smoothies, because then I don't need to add ice; and I can buy frozen berries all year long. If you use fresh berries in this recipe during the summer months, add a few ice cubes as well.

Makes 1 serving

1 cup frozen berries of choice

½ cup plain or vanilla yogurt

¼ cup orange juice

Place berries, yogurt, and juice in the blender. Blend until smooth.

Super Smoothie

FOUNDATION FOODS: Milk, Nuts

When I have leftover ripe bananas, I peel and freeze them. Then I always have a banana on hand to add to smoothies.

Makes 1 serving

¾ cup milk or vanilla soy milk
1 ripe frozen banana
1 tablespoon peanut or almond butter
1 to 2 teaspoons organic chocolate syrup (optional)

Pour the milk (whichever kind you prefer) into the blender, then add the banana, and finally add the nut butter and chocolate syrup. Blend to the desired consistency.

Healthy Popsicles

FOUNDATION FOODS: Berries or Citrus

This recipe is a great use for leftover smoothie ingredients still in the blender! You will need either popsicle molds, or paper cups and popsicle sticks.

The number of servings is variable

100 percent fruit juice such as orange juice, or leftover smoothie
Tiny pieces of fruit (optional)

Pour juice or smoothie into the molds/cups. If desired, add tiny pieces of fresh fruit to each mold. Freeze. If using paper cups, freeze until the mixture is slushy; insert a popsicle stick in the center of each cup when the mixture is stiff enough to hold it in place (but not yet completely solid).

Personalized Trail Mix

FOUNDATION FOODS: Nuts, Whole Grains, Prunes

The possibilities are endless! Let your older toddlers and preschoolers choose their own ingredients; family members can then put their share into resealable containers or plastic bags. Make sure to chop each ingredient to the appropriate size for your child's age (no choking hazards!).

The number of servings is variable

Stick pretzels, chopped or broken into pieces
Dry whole-grain cereal, such as "O" cereal or cereal "squares"
Nuts, finely chopped
Sunflower seeds, shelled
Raisins, dried cranberries, and/or small diced pieces of prunes
Mini-chocolate chips if desired
Graham cracker pieces if desired
Whole-grain crackers, broken into tiny pieces

Place each ingredient into its own small bowl and let the kids create their own trail mix.

Shortcut Guacamole

FOUNDATION FOOD: Avocados

Dr. Tanya uses fresh refrigerated pico de gallo in this extremely easy, healthy recipe.

Makes 4 to 6 servings

2 ripe avocados
½ cup pico de gallo—preferably a fresh, refrigerated variety

Mash the avocado in a small bowl. Add the desired amount of pico de gallo and mix well.

Note: Guacamole turns brown if left out too long. An easy trick to keep the color vibrant is to lightly coat the top of the guacamole with water, then cover with plastic wrap (with the wrap touching the guacamole).

Easy Tortilla/Pita Chips

 **FOUNDATION FOOD: Whole Grains**

Makes 4 to 6 servings

3 whole-wheat tortillas or whole-wheat pitas

⅓ cup olive or canola oil

½ teaspoon salt, or use a salt grinder

⅛ teaspoon ground black pepper, or use a pepper grinder

¼ teaspoon garlic powder, or to taste

Preheat the oven to 400°F. Place a sheet of parchment paper on a baking sheet (optional, for easy cleanup). Stack the tortillas or pitas on top of each other and, using kitchen shears, cut them into triangles (like you are cutting a pie into wedges); or lay the stacked tortillas/pitas on a cutting board and cut them into wedges with a knife. Lay all the pieces flat on the baking sheet and brush them with a thin layer of oil. Turn the pieces over and coat the other side with a thin layer of oil. Generously sprinkle on salt and pepper. (If you don't want to brush the chips, you can toss them in a resealable plastic bag with the oil, then put them on the cookie sheet and add the salt and pepper.) Bake the seasoned chips about 8 to 10 minutes, tossing once. Chips should be light golden and crispy; they will keep getting crispier for a few minutes after cooking. After removing the baking sheet from the oven, sprinkle a little garlic powder on the chips and toss. If you like more flavor, add more garlic powder.

Acknowledgments

If it had not been for my good friend and talented dietitian and chef, Beth Saltz, this book would not be fully cooked nor filled with the flavor that you have hopefully enjoyed. I know that Beth credits her superior cooking skills to her culinary teacher and friend, chef Tim McGrath, and she thanks her husband, Michael, and her adorable daughters, Madison and Zoe, for their endless support.

I would like to thank all of the babies, toddlers, and children I cared for at UCLA, Community Pediatric Medical Group, and Calabasas Pediatrics. You inspired me and taught me how to encourage veggie-loving, no-fuss, healthy-eating kids.

It was only with the assistance of my family and colleagues that my system of Eleven Foundation Foods was developed, harvested, and served. Thank you to my sister, Dr. Candace Katz, an amazing allergist with a vision for a world with fewer food allergies. Also, thank you to Dr. Brynie Collins, my go-to pediatric gastroenterologist, as well as my pediatric support team of fabulous physicians including: Dr. Alanna Levine, Dr. Laura Jana, Dr. Jennifer Shu, Dr. Ari Brown, Dr. Wendy Sue Swanson, Dr. Cara Natterson, Dr. Louise Greenspan, Dr. Nina Shapiro, Dr. Cori Cross, Dr. Meena Taha, Dr. Bhavana Arora, Dr. Jena Liddy, Dr. Angelee Reiner, and Dr. Jessica Hochman. My good friend Dr. Jenn Mann taught me about raising kids to have a healthy relationship with food.

A big thanks to Dr. Leslie Spiegel, who provided many tips and tricks for raising kids with food allergies. Thank you to the team at Community Pediatrics: Dr. Heather Cornett, Dr. David Scherr, Dr. Bill Greene, Dr. Bob Nudelman, and Dr. Howard Goldstine.

For helping to make my new office at Calabasas Pediatrics such a special place, I want to thank Polly Gannon and Angela Beals. Polly's extraordinary nursing and feeding tips educated many moms, including me.

Thank you to Marta Tracy, who introduced me to the team at HarperCollins including Suzanne Wickham, Kathryn Hamilton, Terri Leonard, Amy VanLangen, and Anna Paustenbach—all of whom helped make this book a reality. Kathryn, I could not have published my dream without you. Thank you also to my amazing agent, Alec Shankman, and his dedicated team.

I would not be the person I am today without the guidance and support of my incredible family: my parents, Donald and Louise Remer, who raised me on sprouts and homemade whole-grain bread; my brother, Miles, my on-call tech support; and his wife, Melissa, who taught me invaluable feeding and cooking tips.

Finally, thank you to my husband, Phil, without whom I could not achieve my dreams. We have three wonderful sons—Avrick, Collen, and Maxton—who have taught me more about feeding babies and children than I could ever have learned at the office. My boys constantly surprise me with their willingness to try new foods . . . most of the time.

Notes

Chapter 2: The Program

1. Jessica C. Kiefte-de Jong, Jeanne H. de Vries, Oscar H. Franco et al., "Fish Consumption in Infancy and Asthma-Like Symptoms at Preschool Age," *Pediatrics* 130 (November 2012): 1060–68.
2. G. Biasucci, B. Benenati, L. Morelli et al., "Cesarean Delivery May Affect the Early Biodiversity of Intestinal Bacteria," *Journal of Nutrition* 138, no. 9 (September 2008): 1796S–1800S.
3. Gregory J. Leyer, Shuguang Li, Mohamed E. Mubasher et al., "Probiotic Effects on Cold and Influenza-Like Symptom Incidence and Duration in Children," *Pediatrics* 124, no. 2 (August 1, 2009): e172–e179.
4. M. M. Murphy et al., "Drinking Flavored or Plain Milk Is Positively Associated with Nutrient Intake and Is Not Associated with Adverse Effects on Weight Status in U.S. Children and Adolescents," *Journal of the American Dietetic Association* 108 (2008): 631–39.

Chapter 3: Milk Matters

5. American Academy of Pediatrics, "Breastfeeding and the Use of Human Milk," *Pediatrics* 129, no. 3 (March 1, 2012; published online February 27, 2012): e827–41, doi:10.1542/peds.2011-3552.

Chapter 4: The Infant Program

6. American Academy of Pediatrics, "AAP Offers Advice for Parents Concerned About Arsenic in Food," published online September 6, 2013, https://www.aap.org/en-us/about-the-aap/aap-press-room/pages/AAP-Offers-Advice-For-Parents-Concerned-About-Arsenic-in-Food.aspx.
7. "Arsenic in Your Food," *Consumer Reports,* November 2012, http://www.consumerreports.org/cro/magazine/2012/11/arsenic-in-your-food/index.htm.

8. U.S. Food and Drug Administration, "Questions and Answers: Arsenic in Rice and Rice Products," last modified August 4, 2014, http://www.fda.gov/Food/FoodborneIllnessContaminants/Metals/ucm319948.htm.

Chapter 5: The Toddler Program

9. Ellyn Satter, "The Picky Eater," http://ellynsatterinstitute.org/htf/thepickyeater.php.
10. Dina Rose, *It's Not About the Broccoli: Three Habits to Teach Your Kids for a Lifetime of Healthy Eating* (New York: Penguin, 2014).

Chapter 7: The Modern Family Meal

11. Amber J. Hammons and Barbara H. Fiese, "Is Frequency of Shared Family Meals Related to the Nutritional Health of Children and Adolescents?," published online April 2011, http://pediatrics.aappublications.org/content/early/2011/04/27/peds.2010-1440.short.
12. Matthew W. Gillman et al., "Family Dinner and Diet Quality Among Older Children and Adolescents," *Archives of Family Medicine* 9, no. 3 (2000): 235–40.
13. Bridget Kelly, Becky Freeman, Lesley King et al., "Television Advertising, Not Viewing, Is Associated with Negative Dietary Patterns in Children," *Pediatric Obesity*, doi:10.1111/ijpo.12057; and Tatiana Andreyeva, Inas Rashad Kelly, and Jennifer L. Harris, "Exposure to Food Advertising on Television: Associations with Children's Fast Food and Soft Drink Consumption and Obesity," *Economics & Human Biology* 9 no. 3 (July 2011): 221–33, doi:10:1016/j.ehb.2011.

Chapter 8: Food Allergies and Food Intolerance

14. Kristen Jackson et al., "Trends in Allergic Conditions Among Children: United States, 1997–2011," National Center for Health Statistics Data Brief, 2013, www.cdc.gov/nchs/data/databriefs/db121.htm.
15. Jill A. Poole, Kathy Barriga, Donald Y. M. Leung et al., "Timing of Initial Exposure to Cereal Grains and the Risk of Wheat Allergy," *Pediatrics* 117 no. 6 (June 2006): 2175–82; Bianca E. P. Snijders, Carel Thijs, Ronald van Ree et al., "Age at First Introduction of Cow Milk Products and Other Food Products in Relation to Infant Atopic Manifestations in the First 2 Years of Life: The KOALA Birth Cohort Study," *Pediatrics* 122, no. 1 (July 2008): e115–22; George Du Toit, Yitzhak Katz, Peter Sasieni et al., "Early Consumption of Peanuts in Infancy Is Associated with a Low Prevalence of Peanut Allergy," *Journal of Allergy and Clinical Immunology* 122, no. 5 (November 2008): 984–91; and Jennifer J. Koplin, Nicholas J. Osborne, Melissa Wake et al., "Can Early Introduction of Egg Prevent Egg Allergy in Infants? A Population-Based Study," *Journal of Allergy and Clinical Immunology* 126, no. 4 (October 2010): 807–13.

16. George Du Toit et al., "Randomized Trial of Peanut Consumption in Infants at Risk for Peanut Allergy," *New England Journal of Medicine* 372 (February 26, 2015): 803–13, doi:10.1056/NEJMoa1414850.
17. Stephanie A. Leonard et al., "Dietary Baked Egg Accelerates Resolution of Egg Allergy in Children," *Journal of Allergy and Clinical Immunology* 130 (2012): 473–80, http://www.jacionline.org/article/S0091-6749(12)00953-0/pdf; and Jennifer S. Kim et al., "Dietary Baked Milk Accelerates the Resolution of Cow's Milk Allergy in Children," *Journal of Allergy and Clinical Immunology* 128 (2011): 125–31, http://www.jacionline.org/article/S0091-6749(11)00674-9/pdf.

Chapter 10: Vegetarian and Vegan Kids

18. Louise Greenspan and Julianna Deardorff, *The New Puberty* (New York: Rodale, 2014), 55–56.

Chapter 11: Organic, GMO, and OMG

19. U.S. Environmental Protection Agency, "Agriculture: Organic Farming," last modified September 23, 2015, http://www.epa.gov/agriculture /agriculture-organic-farming.
20. Center for Science in the Public Interest (CSPI), "Going Organic," *Nutrition Action Health Letter,* published online October 2012, https://www.cspinet.org/nah/pdfs /going-organic.pdf.
21. CSPI, "Going Organic."
22. United States Department of Agriculture (USDA), "Meat and Poultry Labeling Terms," last modified August 10, 2015, http://www.fsis.usda.gov/wps/portal/fsis /topics/food-safety-education/get-answers/food-safety-fact-sheets/food-labeling /meat-and-poultry-labeling-terms/meat-and-poultry-labeling-terms.
23. Joel Forman and Janet Silverstein, "Organic Foods: Health and Environmental Advantages and Disadvantages" (AAP clinical report), *Pediatrics* 130, no. 5 (November 1, 2012; published online October 22, 2012), http://pediatrics .aappublications.org/content/130/5/e1406.full.
24. Greenspan and Deardorff, *The New Puberty,* 55–56.
25. L. Charles Bailey et al., "Association of Antibiotics in Infancy with Early Childhood Obesity," *JAMA Pediatrics* 168, no. 11 (November 2014): 1063–69, doi:10.1001 /jamapediatrics.2014.1539.
26. Forman and Silverstein, "Organic Foods," http://pediatrics.aappublications.org /content/130/5/e1406.full.
27. U.S. Food and Drug Administration, "Milk Drug Residue Sampling Survey," March 2015, http://www.fda.gov/downloads/AnimalVeterinary/GuidanceCompliance Enforcement/ComplianceEnforcement/UCM435759.pdf.

28. U.S. Food and Drug Administration, "FDA's Survey of Milk Finds Few Drug Residues," March 5, 2015, http://www.fda.gov/AnimalVeterinary/NewsEvents/CVMUpdates/ucm436379.htm.
29. Miles McEvoy, "Organic 101: The Lifecycle of Organic Food Production," FDA blog entry, April 26, 2012, http://blogs.usda.gov/2012/04/26/organic-101-the-lifecycle-of-organic-food-production/.

Chapter 12: Weighty Issues

30. Yoni Freedhoff, "Why You Shouldn't Put Your Child on a Diet," last modified June 3, 2012, http://www.huffingtonpost.com/yoni-freedhoff/childhood-obesity_b_1399203.html.

Chapter 13: The Feeding Fix

31. Gill Rapley and Tracey Murkett, *Baby-Led Weaning: The Essential Guide to Introducing Solid Foods and Helping Your Baby to Grow Up a Happy and Confident Eater* (New York: The Experiment, 2010).
32. Rapley and Murkett, *Baby-Led Weaning.*
33. Ruth Yaron, *Super Baby Food,* 3rd ed., rev. and updated (Peckville, PA: F. J. Roberts, 2013).
34. Alicia Silverstone, *The Kind Mama: A Simple Guide to Supercharged Fertility, a Radiant Pregnancy, a Sweeter Birth, and a Healthier, More Beautiful Beginning* (New York: Rodale, 2014).
35. Yaron, *Super Baby Food.*
36. Silverstone, *The Kind Mama.*
37. Silverstone, *The Kind Mama.*
38. Massachusetts General Hospital, "Delayed Introduction to Gluten Appears Not to Prevent Celiac Disease in At-Risk Infants," *ScienceDaily,* October 1, 2014, www.sciencedaily.com/releases/2014/10/141001185750.htm.
39. Missy Chase Lapine, *The Sneaky Chef: Simple Strategies for Hiding Healthy Foods in Kids' Favorite Meals* (Philadelphia: Running Press, 2007); and Jessica Seinfeld, *Deceptively Delicious: Simple Secrets to Get Your Kids Eating Good Food* (New York: William Morrow, 2010).

Chapter 14: The Picky Eater

40. Rachel Goldman, Cynthia Radnitz, and Robert E. McGrath, "The Role of Family Variables in Fruit and Vegetable Consumption in Preschool Children," *Journal of Public Health Research* 1, no. 2 (June 15, 2012; published online May 15, 2012): 143–48, doi:10.4081/jphr.2012.e22.

Index